WHAT PEOPLE ARE SAYING
ABOUT "QUIET MIRACLES"

Sid Levinsohn, a local pharmacist and medical researcher, has become a nationally known expert on the topic of surviving chronic and terminal illnesses."

    – *StarTribune*, April 22, 2002

It's a book for those who yearn to think outside of the box and to discover their potential as creators. If you ever found yourself looking for the answers, the edict "Thinking makes it so!" speaks volumes about our personal ability to create the kind of life we thought was unattainable. Read carefully, as every word is a gem.

    – Christine Traxler M.D.

Congratulations for being selected as one of Minnesota's Champions of Health. It's quite an honor to be nominated by members of your community and to be selected by an independent panel of judges from across the state for your work to improve the health of Minnesota— one community at a time.

    – Mark W. Banks, M.D.
    President and CEO, BlueCross BlueShield

The seminar made a world of difference. It helped me come to terms with my illness and helped in finding a sense of peace.

    – Cindy Hilger, WCCO-TV

You are a wonderful speaker with a great message. I found it fascinating to listen to your facts and stories and heard similar comments from other participants.

    – Maria Falcone, American Cancer Society

Thank you again for your hard work and the tremendous job you did in your workshop. The participants gave very positive comments and I was pleased with the way you were able to give each one special attention. This is unheard of in a workshop setting.

    – Maureen Hoberg, R.N.,
    Ridgeview Medical Center

I can't tell you how many times you and your wonderful session come to mind. You are a very special person whom God is using in a wonderful way.

> – Char Jorgensen,
> BlueCross BlueShield of Minnesota

We would like to express our appreciation for your inspiring presentation, Quiet Miracles during the 3rd annual Fall Education Summit, Treatment Challenges in the Continuum of Care.

> – The Rev. Peter Lundholm and The Rev. Linda S. Campbell,
> Chaplains, Department of Veterans Affairs Medical Center.

Sid brings his professional background as a pharmacist, combined with his own personal experience as a cancer survivor, into every session he leads. Perhaps more importantly, he brings his optimism, support, and enthusiasm to help patients, family members, friends, and caregivers deal with cancer and other chronic illnesses. He is able to push people beyond their normal boundaries while respecting individual differences and abilities.

> – Jerry Waldman, Executive Director, JFCS

Your workshops were the highlight of the year.

> Gina and Stan Kugler, workshop attendees

I wanted to share a few thoughts about your workshop…by saying you are an amazing human being with an extraordinary gift of giving. There wasn't a single individual in the room who wasn't touched by your work, your words. Your message was strong and clear, gentle and embracing.

> – Debra Levenstein,
> Director, Family Life Education

Thank you for agreeing to do [Quiet Miracles]. I hope you will consider returning to our community and helping us with this important educational journey.

> – Beverly Propes,
> R.N. and Public Health Consultant, Pilot City Health

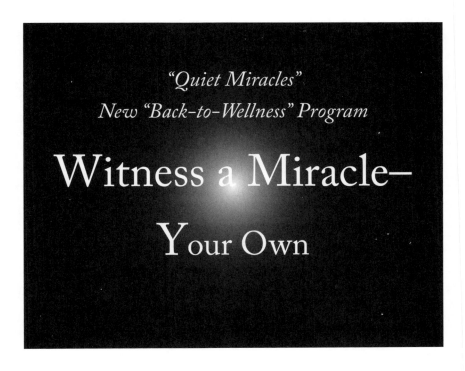

"Quiet Miracles"
New "Back-to-Wellness" Program

Witness a Miracle–
Your Own

The Fastest Way to
Turn Your Life and Health Around!
12 NEW Scientific Discoveries
That Can Slow Down, Stop and Even Reverse
Serious Illness—Naturally!

Sidney H. Levinsohn, R.Ph.

NODIN PRESS

The information, recommendations, and material in this book are for reference and guidance only and are not intended to be a medical guide or manual for self-treatment or a substitute for a physician's diagnosis and care. The editors urge anyone with continuing medical problems or symptoms to consult a qualified physician, since this information is not intended as a substitute for any treatment prescribed by your doctor.

ISBN 13: 978-1-932472-63-9

Library of Congress Cataloging-in-Publication Data

Levinsohn, Sidney H.
  Witness a miracle-your own : the fastest way to turn your life and health around! : 12 new scientific discoveries that can slow down, stop and even reverse serious illness-naturally! / Sidney H. Levinsohn.
     p. cm.
  "Quiet Miracles New Back-to-Wellness Program."
  ISBN 978-1-932472-63-9
  1. Alternative medicine. 2. Visualization. 3. Mental suggestion. I. Title.
RC49.L4385 2007
616.001'9--dc22
                          2007031956

Nodin Press is a division of Micawber's, Inc.
530 N. Third Street,
Suite 120.
Minneapolis, MN 55401

Acknowledgements

Many people have helped me to make this book a reality, and it has been my priviledge to work with them. A number of the fellow travelers I have met on my medical journey have become friends, and they have taught me volumes about self-healing and the unity of life in the best possible way—through their words and actions. They helped me discover what life means and how it should be lived. For the same reason, my eternal thanks go out also to my mother and father, Dorothy and Max Levinsohn, whose message and spirit taught me to challenge many of the commonplace stereotypes.

This book was written with unconditional love for my family and those who attend my Quiet Miracles workshops. Several chapters were created with my granddaughter Erica in mind. If she is ever faced with a crisis and things seem darkest and draining, I'd like her to entertain the possibility that everything in life is possible, if you believe it is. (Are you listening, honey? If you don't read this book and practice its daily sustenance, I'll come back as a friendly ghost to remind you!). As well, the book is intended for Andrew, Noah and Haylee, and future grandchildren, so they will never ever hesitate to brazenly buck conventional wisdom and think for themselves. My advice, as they have so often heard, is that to change the world for the better, you must begin to change your own framework of thoughts and feelings. Only you possess the creative power to trigger this change.

The book is intended also for use by my loving sons Craig and Loren, and their spouses, Rachel and Shari, when they want to buck the system or rid themselves of toxic beliefs and engage in raucous fun—which I heartily recommend on a regular basis.

To my entire family I offer this counsel: Be active idealists— against the current if need be. Be a force for good. Believe in uncovering each person's basic good intent and you will discover it. Keep always in mind that each of us is given the inner power to use our potential as a developing spiritual being to make each day a purposeful adventure. Yoda in The Empire Strikes Back said it best: "Do or do not. There is no try!"

What will linger forever and always in my memory is the deep sensitivity and love of my wife Joanie Levinsohn. Her monumental love and concern helped me to shake my fist at cancer and fulfill my destiny. Few ever find in a lifetime what I found with Joanie—resolve and smooth passage in a challenging world.

I also wish to thank the Founding Father of Quiet Miracles Stuart Friedell and the initial support team he assembled of Bob Stillman, Marvin Stillman, Marshall Lifson, Ralph Stillman and Norman Winer. Also, a special word of gratitude to Christine Traxler, M.D., Jerri Johnson, Alan Hymes, M.D, Jerry Brill, John Levin, Margie Weil, Jim Peterson, Steve Lear, the blessed memory of Judy Silverman and Elaine Leff, Norton Stillman of Nodin Press, John Toren, Rena St. Cyr and many other supporting friends for lifting more than a finger to elevate the Quiet Miracles Program and this book.

– Sid Levinsohn

Write to: Quiet Miracles
4122 Black Oaks Lane North
Plymouth, Minnesota 55446
Phone: 763-519-0592
 Email: Quietmiracles@comcast.net
Website: endhealthworries.com

For appearances or workshops by Sid Levinsohn, contact Quiet Miracles at 763-579-0592 or email quietmiracles@comcast.net.

Contents

Foreword

I met Sid Levinsohn briefly when I was a premed student at the University of Minnesota in 1940. Thirty-six years later, our paths crossed again and we discovered that we both had been practicing meditative techniques for many years and shared many common interests. Seasoned by many similar life experiences, we renewed and deepened our friendship.

Sid has many wonderful and brilliantly insightful facets to his personality. He is one of the smartest people I know and a keen observer of human nature. He approaches the totality of life with a calm, curious fascination. He tackles adverse events as a personal challenge and sees in them the opportunity to understand life's lessons and to learn and grow. He is a man intent on turning life's lemons into lemonade.

In his book, Sid describes his self-healing journey and the lessons he learned from talking to long-term cancer survivors during his bout with cancer and conducting workshops for those with chronic illnesses. Out of these experiences, he has created a transformational "blueprint" developed for coping and overcoming the disease — a strategy that will, in all likelihood, help him remain a long-term cancer survivor himself. The step-by-step techniques that he developed from his research and interviews are so simple that anyone can learn them.

As Sid reveals in his writings, his interest in nontraditional healing practices has given him valuable information too often ignored by our healthcare system. When combined, the unconventional and conventional medical systems offer a holistic approach to successful healing. Sid asserts that if practiced faithfully, result-oriented mental visualization (where healing first takes place), can rid the body of abnormal cells. Sid's purpose in writing about his healing journey is to give a message of hope to others. In his own words, he says, "This book provides the reader a clear, empowering formula that can pave the way to your taking charge of your own healing journey."

As a physician, I've observed firsthand the benefit of a positive mental outlook in patients coping with a serious disease. Yet the practice of self-healing imagery to initiate and sustain a physiologic process that can result in the destruction of abnormal cells runs counter to conventional scientific and medical wisdom. However, as Sid points out, scores of physicians are becoming open to using some unorthodox therapies, in light of anecdotal testimonies to their success.

Still, the very idea that mental imagery could actually harness external or internal energy forces to help the body destroy abnormal cells would be absolutely rejected as "hocus pocus" by the vast majority of medical scientists and allopathic physicians. But I know Sid Levinsohn. He's sincere and he's credible. If mental imagery and the healing factors he describes worked for him and long-term cancer survivors, I want to know more.

As a medical specialist in general thoracic (chest) and vascular surgery, I always practiced within the orthodox standards of my specialties. During my training, I was involved in clinical investigations of the effects of chemotherapeutic agents in patients with terminal cancer, as well as in experimental surgical projects in animals. As a product of Western scientific culture and methods, I believed in the scientific method, which states basically that for something to be accepted as true, it must satisfy the scientific principles of study. In addition, experiments and testing have to produce statistically significant results. Therefore, if an event under study is predictable by statistics and repeated verification, it is deemed true. On the other hand, if results of a study or elements of experience are not of statistical significance, or if they cannot be reproduced, they are considered untrue.

Deep down, I was troubled by this narrow definition of truth. For example, suppose you tell me that you often dream in color and I reply, "Prove it or else it simply isn't true." Does my statement make your dreams less colorful?

Fully steeped in the scientific culture, I became rigid and "hard-nosed." Incidentally, I was also an agnostic. Well, one day while "traveling to Damascus," I had a very personal experience. Firsthand, I suddenly realized that mental telepathy, telekinesis (moving objects either directly or from a remote distance by thought process) and other paranormal phenomena, were not necessarily fairy tales, but real. My scientific paradigm was instantly shattered. I was depressed for days, until I had a sudden awe-inspiring realization that the universe is unbelievably more complicated and wonderful than science could validly establish by evidence or demonstration. I concluded that the accepted paradigm or archetype of scientific investigation required a radical redefinition. For me, agnosticism had to go. Truly, there was a magnificent God. Today, I consider myself a "holistic" physician.

All of us have experiences or heard of events that appear to have no logical or scientific explanation, so we call them coincidences. Yet, they seem to happen rather regularly, which leaves us wondering whether all these "accidental" occurrences are not somehow connected. Can they be the result of the same kind of energy force? Can mental imagery focus these energies to conquer other life-threatening diseases? I suspect so.

How many of us have witnessed the astonishing healing power of prayer? I have observed that when we pray alone or as a group, happy outcomes that beat the odds against conventional wisdom happen far more commonly than one would expect by chance alone. Yet, the tendency to pass off the results as a coincidence rather than viewing them as a miracle is all too common.

Do we subliminally communicate with each other through these energies via a sixth sense? How many of us have been thinking about a friend or close relative, and several hours later have received a call from him or her?

Not long ago, I saw a human-interest TV program that related a remarkable story. A U.S. Army serviceman, when stationed in Thailand years ago, had a son with a Thai woman. A few years after his return to the United States, the serviceman lost contact with the boy. Not long ago, for some unknown reason, he felt compelled to stop at a neighborhood convenience store for gasoline, even though he had never stopped there before. When he went inside to pay the bill, the clerk recognized his name on the credit card. After the clerk asked several leading questions, they discovered that they were father and son!

The inherent energy forces obviously used by the long-term cancer survivors described in Sid's book are not considered energy by traditional physicists. About 20 years ago, I had the pleasure of meeting Dr. Otto Schmidt, a world-renowned physicist and professor emeritus of biophysics at the University of Minnesota. Dr. Schmidt has written hundreds of scientific articles and lectured worldwide. He is the creator of hundreds of inventions, including the three-dimensional electrocardiogram and the Schmidt Trigger, a very rapid electrical switching system without which all modern computers could not function.

During one of our conversations, I asked him about his thoughts regarding mental telepathy and psychokinesis. He said that if these phenomena were real, the basic tenets of physics would have to be altered. His response, surprisingly, was that he believed such phenomena exist. Michael Crichton, author of *Jurassic Park* and a graduate of Harvard Medical School, has also written *Travels*, a book in which he reveals his real-life experiences in exploring many different psychic practices and avenues of paranormal activities — similar in nature to the healing miracle Sid describes in this book. In the final chapter of his book, Crichton summarizes his thoughts and poses the questions he would like to ask scientists regarding paranormal phenomena. I highly recommend that this book be required reading for all first-year medical students.

Sid Levinsohn may appear to some to be presenting exercises in wishing, while awaiting his death from cancer. However, I believe the real truth of the matter is that he has laid out a formula that actually links to a source of internal healing energy, which is accessible to all. By using Sid's techniques, anyone has the potential to become a long-term cancer survivor. I personally believe that the healing energy exhibited by those who defy all scientific odds is part of creation that stems from God in part or in whole. Be that as it may, the practical self-healing practices described by Sid can work for virtually all patients, regardless of their personal beliefs or religious preferences. After all, mind and body are not separate entities, but one. For proof, simply ask long-term cancer survivors. Who among us can argue with their success?

To those of you reading this book who have a life-threatening disease, my best healing prayers go out to you. May this book give you a way to stay hopeful and retain a vision of a healthy outcome. I am reminded of an ancient proverb that says a happy heart is good medicine and a cheerful mind can work wondrous healing. In all areas of healing, combining that advice with conventional medicine may be the best science of all.

Willfully stay happy and healthy!

– Alan Hymes, M D

Chapter One

What Everyone Ought to Know About Making "Miracles"

"The spirit is the life, the mind is the builder,
and the physical is the result."

– Edgar Cayce

Have you ever given serious thought to phenomena for which science has no suitable explanation? Here are just a few such conundrums:

- How can people with multiple personality disorder exhibit different chronic illnesses depending upon which personality is present?

- How are some cancer patients able to incite the mind to alter a life-threatening illness?

- How is it that actors playing comedy roles can have a different immune system response than those performing a depressing drama?

- How can benign placebos, prescribed by physicians, sometimes prove markedly effective?

- How is it that students who believe they can control their immune system response can increase or decrease the activity of neutrophil white blood cells in their blood stream?

- How can subjects under hypnosis perform extraordinary physical feats?

- How can some people walk unscathed on a bed of blistering coals?

- How is it that miners trapped underground, with only one hour of oxygen, are still alive when found and dug out long afterward.? (The sole exception: the one miner with a watch, who was intentionally misleading the others when they repeatedly asked the time remaining, and the only one aware that the hour had passed.)

- How is it that medical students often experience symptoms of diseases they study?

- How can migraine sufferers effectively manage their health using biofeedback training?

- How is it that a healthy tribal member, given a voodoo "hex" by a witch doctor, soon dies even though he shows no evidence of disease?

The surprising answers to these questions, and how you can achieve your own "miracle," is what this book is going to show you.

L et's start by discussing self-suggestive beliefs, which can be a powerful force for activating the conditions described above. Such beliefs made it possible for Japanese Kamikaze pilots to carry out suicide missions during World War II, and the same intense emotions are at work today among those seeking martyrdom in the Middle East and elsewhere. On the other hand, many people who have chronic illnesses sommon the same enegery, but direct it, not toward self-sacrifice, but in the opposite direction, toward feelings of hopelessness and helplessness. Such highly suggestive beliefs generate vivid mental pictures that appear quite logical and justifiable to the receptive mind. That is to say, beliefs have an energetic life all of their own.

"You are the maker of yourself," said philosopher James Allen. According to Allen and many other philosophers, our purpose in life is to learn how to be responsible shapers of life experiences through the creative power of belief and thought.

> **Your outer world is formed by the beliefs and thoughts that you choose to accept as "truth."**

This central declaration can be further summarized in three words: *Outside matches inside*; better yet, *Beliefs become real(ity)*. What you intensely picture and emotionally concentrate on internally comes into existence externally. It you don't nurture mental images and thoughts of wellness, it will be difficult to become well. The picture-forming power of your mind has more creative capacity for healing than you have ever imagined. But to tap into this inner realm of power will require that you push beyond the comfortable boundaries of your current beliefs and thoughts, which can often be self-limiting.

The Law of Attraction

Your thoughts are like a magnet that attracts to itself all within its sphere of activity. In short, like attracts like. Mental images and thoughts of wellness attract wellness. Thoughts of illness and decrepitude have the opposite effect. Think positive thoughts and concentrated wellness energy flows toward you. Think self-defeating thoughts and wellness energy flows away from you. The powerful energy of optimism adds to your strength, while negative mental images weaken the body's natural healing defenses. To become stronger and heal, you need to defuse and overcome negative emotional images that block and delay wellness. Long-term cancer survivors prove that nothing can draw wellness to them like the power (intensity) of belief coupled with positive mental imagery.

The Law of Attraction and Expectation works in everyday ways as well. Let me give you an example:

Patients with Multiple Personality Disorder(MPD) exhibit different organic conditions when acting out different personalities. Each time a different personality surfaces, there is a corresponding change in the response of the immune system. For example, and individual with MPD might exhibit serious diabetes, yet one hour later, when another personality has appeared, all signs of diabetes vanish.

One day, wanting to learn more about the subject of MPD, I resolved to pay a visit to the University of Minnesota Medical School Library. My wife Joanie mentioned that a local discount operator was having a half-price sale on books, and she asked if I would care to accompany her. I explained my research project to her and said that I would really prefer to pass. It then occurred to me that the discount store was near the medical library, so I told Joanie I would be happy to join her after all, and off we went.

As it happened, the library had just closed, so we headed directly to the discount store. Wandering aimlessly among some 25,000 books, I found that my thoughts remained intensely focused on the subject of MPD. Within a few moments, almost magically, I reached for a book entitled *Act Now*. I had no idea why I was drawn to this particular book. Certainly I had little interest in theatrical performance, which is what the book appeared to be about. Still, for some deeper reason, I found myself compelled to purchase that particular book. Arriving home, I flipped open the pages and there, staring me in the face, was virtually everything I wanted to know about multiple personality disorder. Would you believe I had even opened the book to the exact page on the subject?

Coincidence? Perhaps. Yet it seems to me that such coincidences—events without apparent connection—take place far too often to fit that convenient explanation. Simply put, I believe that we attract such events to ourselves. My belief is that the causal agent underlying the properties of coincidence can be defined as the workings of the unlimited creative power of the subconscious in league with its working partner—the Law of Attraction.

Here are several more examples: One day I was scheduled to give a speech to a group of nurses at a local medical center. When I arrived at the appointed time, I was told that the previous speaker was running a bit late. While waiting in the reading room, I found myself attracted to a year-old magazine with an article on psychic phenomenon. I paged quickly to the article and was soon absorbed in the subject matter. Unfortunately, before I could finish reading the story, I was called upon to make my presentation. During the talk, I had difficulty concentrating on anything but that captivating article.

Completing my talk late, and hurrying to get to another appointment, I had no time to read the remaining portion of the article. I gave serious thought to simply taking the magazine—it was already a year old; nobody would miss it—but decided not to, reasoning that I could return later and make a copy of the article I had found so fascinating.

When I arrived home that evening, the very first thing my wife said to me was, "Honey, I was at the hairdresser's today and saw a magazine with an article I just knew you would love, so I asked my beautician if I could take it home. Since it was a year old, he said, 'No problem.'"

There, in her hand, was the object of my thoughts.

Invariably, when I'm looking for a solution to a particular problem, I quite literally take it to bed with me with the expectation that, through the Law of Attraction, the answer will somehow appear when I awaken. Often, while I'm shaving or taking a shower the next morning, the solution appears. I'm to the point now, when using a pre-sleep suggestion approach (explained in detail later), I expect answers to arrive from my inner senses on the following morning.

Let your slogan be:
"I Can, I Will, I Dare, I Do!"

The Law of Attraction and Expectation is an efficient and dependable creative force that can be controlled and directed. When I'm searching for information about a particular subject, like MPD, the desired information customarily comes to me from multiple sources, such as e-mail messages, publications, a letter, you name it—providing the exact information I am seeking. I'm convinced this has a great deal to do with (a) my having an explorative and receptive mental attitude, and (b) the core belief that I personally have a hand in realizing my strong desires.

To further illustrate my point, one day I was discussing with a friend an idea regarding a key phrase—"How to take the "t" out of can't!" I was looking to incorporate the slogan into an upcoming speech that would revolve around the central theme of the Law of Attraction. My friend, who knew nothing about the subject, offered to lend me a book he had not yet read, although it had been in his library for many years. The name of the book: *The*

Inner Secret by Edward E. Beals. The volume proved to be a truly excellent primer. I believe that it was no accident that Beale's key phrase for tapping into the power of the mind was quite similar to my own. His slogan of choice: "I Can, I Will, I Dare, I Do!"

The Law of Attraction does not necessarily require such conscious direction, however. During my college years, for example, I took several medical courses dealing with the symptoms of acute diseases, and a number of students actually began to manisfest the physical symptoms of the diseases we were studying. This response is similar in some ways to the dynamic action of a placebo prescribed by a physician, which prove to be remarkably effective though it "does" nothing. (The placebo phenomena will be discussed in greater detail in a later chapter.) In both cases, individuals are being emotionally and physically drawn to the condition they happen to be "thinking" about—in the first case disease, in the second case wellness. Open to suggestion, they fail to realize that the emerging physical symptoms are their own personal creation.

Putting the Law of Attraction to work for you 24 hours a day

In Appendix II you'll find a prayer/dream exercise describing how you can make use of your dreams to restore your health, thus putting the Law of Attraction to work for you around the clock. Just prior to sleep, and in the morning before fully waking, are the most favorable times for indelibly anchoring such self-suggestions. Make sure your thought-suggestions are clear and precise so the subconscious can carry out the results you desire. Keep reinforcing your suggestions after you awaken, trusting your body's inherent processes, and you'll be astonished by the results you attract to yourself.

The sum total of your past beliefs and thoughts have led you to the path you currently are on. You are, today, the aggregate of yesterday's choices. By the same logic, the thoughts you summons *today* will form tomorrow's life experience. Thinking of life as a learning process attracts soul growth (it is my belief that all of us are here for a purpose—or nothing has a purpose).

It's become apparent to me through my interviews with long-term cancer survivors that they have drawn wellness to themselves by uncovering the following prescription for wellness:

- Persistently visualizing mental pictures of your desired goal as certainty,

- backed by belief, feelings (live vibrating energy) and positive self-talk, and

- when acted upon by an impressionable subconscious mind,

- sets in active motion, the Law of Attraction,

- which bolsters the body's defense system.

Highly suggestive mental conditioners

Ever wonder why slogan stores are successful? Why you see catchy phrases on the walls and desks of successful people? Why motivational speakers wrap their messages around a well-turned catch phrase? Highly suggestive words serve as steady reminders and emotional conditioners to help you tap into the mind's full potential and overcome feelings of powerlessness. Such reminders give us a better awareness of the necessity for concentration and mental repetition, preventing despairing thoughts from crippling our lives. I have had a declaration by philosopher William Ward on my office wall for many years that sums up the mechanics of my basic life outlook. I must have read it hundreds of times. It says simply:

If you can imagine it, you can achieve it.
If you can dream it, you can become it.

Still think you're powerless to orchestrate your subjective world with positive mental images, thoughts and feelings? Let me give you another example:

One day I was paying bills and doing assorted monthly tasks that I dislike when I decided to ease the tension by tuning in to a radio station that played music from the Fifties. Almost immediately, I felt mentally revitalized. In an effort to continue livening up my pensive frame of mind, I decided to play a few CDs featuring Pete Fountain, Oscar Peterson, and my all-time favorite, Errol Garner. I then played my favorite comedy tape. There I sat, taking a little Zen-like respite, all the while smiling and wondering what could be sweeter than paying bills? Honestly, I can't ever remember laughing out loud and feeling so good while paying my bills.

Who would have believed it? What was going on?

The process of spurring the Law of Attraction into action involves planting the right kind of thoughts and feelings into your mind, habitually fortifying yourself with strong self-talk and affirmative thought-forms (mental pictures in your mind's eye), and imagining your goal as *already achieved*. It's also good to remember that the stronger the intensity of your mental imagery, the sooner the Law of Attraction will come into play. The meaning is clear: you have to "show up" (consciously take action) to make yourself better. This will involve identifying the core beliefs that form the framework of your existence—the rules you've chosen to live your life by—and replacing those that are negative in orientation with the renewed energy of outcome-oriented visualization, focused belief, good feelings, high intention (the underdog's "fighting spirit"), and trust in your inherent creative power. In short, you need a point-by-point "Wellness Action Plan" to experience self-empowerment and a sense of congruity with Divine Energy Source. This guide will show you how to make and follow such a plan.

The key is to change your toxic thoughts and feelings while creating strong, repeated mental images that generate a back-to-wellness mentality.

Let's talk more about the power of belief, thoughts, and feelings, and the wellness frame of mind it creates. It's important to understand that you attract to yourself the life circumstance on which you repeatedly focus your picture-making imagination. Creating strong mental images of wellness, backed by the power of strong belief and emotional energy, acts upon the subconscious mind and mobilizes the Law of Attraction.

Controlled experiments have demonstrated that athletes who regularly practice mental imagery and positive feelings perform better than those who do not. There is no question of the importance of creating clear and sustaining vivid mental images of the outcome you strongly desire. To automatically trigger the Law of Attraction, it's important *you clearly imagine, and register in detail*, the emotional *intensity* of your mental images of wellness, imagining them as *naturally* a part of your body.

In his book, *Conscious Autosuggestion*, French psychologist Emile Coue tells a story about Michelangelo who had just completed a statue:

"You have been idle since I last saw you," said a friend.

"By no means," responded Michelangelo. "I have softened this feature, brought out this muscle; I have given more expressions to the lips and more energy to the limb."

"Well," said his friend, "but all these are trifles."

"It may be so," said Michelangelo, "but recollect that trifles make perfection, and perfection is no trifle."

The key to setting the Law of Attraction in motion can be stated in one short sentence:

Your deeply rooted beliefs are the rules you live by!

If you think about it, positive belief—a highly concentrated form of actualizing energy—is the chief factor behind remarkable barrier-breaking performances. Roger Bannister broke the four-minute mile. Sir Edmund Hillary ascended Mount Everest. Helen Keller lived a life of achievement, despite being divested of sight, hearing and speech. Strong beliefs that set off the Law of Attraction can create acts of incredible accomplishment. By the same token, deeply embedding diseased beliefs and defective thoughts in your subconscious mind can attract ill-health.

Your core beliefs and thoughts self-hypnotically speak to the cells in your body. If your mind is fed self-destructive beliefs and mental images, a chain reaction sets in motion the Law of Attraction. Your feelings change. As a repercussion, your body's ability to reverse disease diminishes. Since your physical body is the living picture of your beliefs and feelings, it follows that what materializes physically mirrors the mental pictures and emotion you have created. This is reason enough to turn your focus to what can go right in your life, biologically and otherwise. When circumstances are off-center, start thinking like Thomas Edison, who said that once he knew what didn't work, he was that much closer to finding what would.

> *They who conquer believe they can.*
> – Ralph Waldo Emerson

Like a furnace that throws off heat, the Law of Attraction triggers physical experience. If you center your imagination on pictures of fear, for example, your entire biological framework will be affected. This, in turn, will elicit feelings of helplessness and hopelessness. How often have you encountered a stressful situation and been seized by a headache or stomach distress? When was the last time your narrow perceptions caused you to feel depressed and to act as if you were powerless, producing a biochemical reaction that eventually blocked energy needed by your immune system? The emotions that creep into your body as a result of harmful beliefs are chemicals, after all, and viewing the world through a negative lens of anger, victim consciousness, or some other unresolved emotional issues will precipitate hormonal changes that can be corrosive. Your thoughts have live energy. You alone determine if the energy you're sending to your body is positive or negative.

Cultivate your mental belief-garden.

Here is an apt analogy for describing the Law of Attraction and Expectation and other definitive laws of nature: Imagine yourself planting mental wellness seedlings in the form of positive beliefs and feelings (envisioning them as living organisms) in the rich soil of your psyche. Know that in due time, these powerful seedlings will take root, restoring you to emotional and physical well-being. Look upon your new healthy belief seedlings as ones you strongly desire to flower, bringing you new positive experiences that you cannot wait to bring to fruition.

Take charge of your medical journey and life.

Since your body is altered physically by your beliefs and thoughts, begin to consciously picture yourself as the controller of your life circumstances, not the thing being controlled. Trust your own inherent abilities. Inoculate your mind with belief seedlings that prevent despair from taking root, since such implanting lowers the body's natural defenses. Tell yourself that choosing to take the path of discouragement is unsafe and self-destructive. Make a profound effort to repeat the picture-forming suggestion that you are a creator of your life experiences and can naturally attract wellness via the Law of Attraction. Soon your cumulative mental images will begin to incite the powerful subconscious to alter your mental and physical condition. Be receptive, persistent, expectant, and optimistic.

Beliefs can make us prisoners.

Negative suggestions believed intensely with strong feeling may become habitual beliefs, thoughts and internal dialogue (self-talk). Taken for truth and left unexamined, those negative beliefs become a rigid attitude of mind that may manifest in poor health and/or adverse life experiences. As it is, many negative suggestions, firmly implanted in adolescence, give rise to unyielding beliefs which continue to evade inspection into maturity. There are numerous examples of detrimental beliefs that if directly ingrained in children can endure well into adulthood:

"If you have a headache, take an aspirin."

"If you're depressed, call the doctor for a prescription."

"Heart attacks run in our family."

"You have panic attacks just like your mother."

"Cancer is usually fatal."

"Without good grades, there's no way you're going to make it in life."

"If you don't get enough sleep, you'll get sick."

"Stomach trouble? You're probably constipated!"

"Can't sleep? Take a sleeping pill."

"You're too self-conscious. You'll probably always be the bashful type."

"You're always nervous about something. I don't see you ever changing."

Think illness—attract and realize illness!

Taking adverse judgements and suggestions like these to heart can disturb healthy cells and already weakened vital organs. Children who receive such specific and incisive suggestions from those in authority are, in effect, being hypnotized. Youngsters typically accept such negative beliefs without scrutiny, and thus unknowingly lay the groundwork for the negativity that can undermine health later in life.

On the opposite end of the spectrum are long-term cancer survivors who, because they make a commitment to practice positive outcome-oriented visual imagery, enable themselves to unite body, mind and spirit for a far healthier life. My own experience interviewing cancer survivors and conducting workshops for people with chronic illnesses has convinced me that those who persistently practice and regularly reinforce the immense power of self-suggestion, confidently acting as if their mental imagery is already achieved, can set into motion the Law of Attraction which effectively strengthens the body's natural healing process.

Act as if you *can* take the "t" out of can't

Flash pictures of wellness on your mental screen, focusing and acting as if those images are already achieved, and emotional energy will become increasingly accessible, thus validating that mental imagery. On the other hand, if you repeatedly summon unhealthy mental pictures—a high-wire act with no visible net—you're almost certain to disrupt your health. The challenge is daring, every day, to act as if the impossible is not only possible but is already a "fact" of life. Remind yourself that Infinite Energy is within. Dare to call upon it to set off the Law of Attraction. What harm can it do? I would rather be downright sorry for what I tried, than for what I failed to try.

The universal law at work is this: You are most likely to get what you focus your attention on. Like a mirror image, this reflects your firmly accepted cluster of beliefs and thoughts.

We are ever in the Presence of an Infinite and
Eternal Energy from which all things proceed.
– Herbert Spencer

Awakening your consciousness to wellness requires learning to let repeated vibrations (live, flowing energy) of mental imagery, confident expectation and emotional persistence dominate your thoughts. Taking vigorous action by following the "12 powerful back-to-wellness exercises" prescribed in Appendix II will quickly set off the impressive force of Infinite Energy and the Law of Attraction, bringing a new inner sense of self-empowerment into your life. Remember, it is infinitely important that YOU play an active role in the creation of wellness.

And don't underestimate the ability of your creative imagination to alter your toxic beliefs and feelings, awakening a healing giant. Concentrating your inner dimension on the "Wellness Action Plan" outlined in Appendix III will intuitively expand your scope of mental activity, thus inciting the great Law of Attraction into action. There is no need to take my word for this, nor do I ask that you agree with my basic premise. Follow the self-discovery suggestions step-by-step, and you'll prove to yourself that you *can* tap into Infinite Energy, the source of all remarkable occurrences.

How do YOU define the limits of what you can achieve?

Be honest: Are you underestimating your inherent Infinite Energy within—that vast reservoir of universal energy that can attract and accelerate healing? You must understand that you and Infinite Energy are one. What's more, this energy is freely available. You can draw upon it at any time by focusing on whatever you consciously believe and, mentally picturing it with strong feeling and an inner knowing. If you practice this method persistently, your subconscious mind will tap into Infinite Energy and set off the Law of Attraction, and the vibrations of your focused thoughts, feelings, and intent will attract matching events into your life.

But to do this effectively, it's important that you clear away old toxic feelings that are exerting negative influence by tracing them back to their roots in old wounds and hurts (beliefs) and replacing them with mental images of wellness, using the outcome-oriented visual imagery techniques that I've been describing.

On the next page is self-dialogue that can attract health and energy to the very core of your being:

Each day, I get what my dominating thoughts focus on. I need to realize that I only accept thoughts that fit my basic beliefs (positive or negative). Others are either consciously or unconsciously rejected. I may need to remind myself often that positive thoughts cause healing energy to flow smoothly throughout my physical body, while negative thoughts impede healing. Truly, I am my thoughts. Since I literally "act out" my beliefs, thoughts and expectations, I need to pay special attention to which thoughts I welcome, and which will adversely affect my immune response. Each day, I need to get in the habit of deconstructing the obstacle—beliefs, really—that stand in the way of the outcome I strongly desire and visually picture as already achieved. My physical challenge is there to remind me of the toxic belief behind it. The challenge will likely disappear when I clear up the toxic belief. I need to remember I can only change what's without from within.

Thinking deeply about the set of illuminating questions below can help you begin to redefine what you believe is possible.

Below are a number of leading questions to ask yourself. They encourage you to examine the destructive thoughts you send yourself daily that may affect your body's basic defense mechanisms. Honest responses will assist you in focusing your awareness away from the tyranny of old beliefs that reinforce limitations, delay resolution, and impede both physical healing and spiritual growth.

- Do I give myself the *freedom to explore the nature of my mind* in order to learn what thoughts and feelings I am most prone to focusing my attention on?

- Do I ever ask myself what harmful messages I'm sending to myself that I do need to change?"

- Do I have the courage to examine the rigid beliefs, thoughts, expectations and feelings I've programmed myself to perceive, understanding that they define who I am?

- Am I aware that the new science is suggesting that *there is no reality until it is perceived reality?* In other words, if I don't perceive wellness, abundance, etc., I will not create it. I can create only events I perceive.

- Since I can't surpass my own self-definition, in what ways have I chosen to limit my perception of what is actually possible?

- Do I generally listen to and follow what my intuition is telling me?

- Do I find myself preoccupied with feelings of hopelessness and helplessness, unable to squeeze *new good-feeling thoughts* into the structure of my old, toxic beliefs?

- Do I recognize that my core beliefs and expectations direct the state of health and vitality of every cell and vital organ in my body?

- Have I made up my mind to alter my self-limiting beliefs, or have I unconditionally surrendered to the belief that what will be, will be?

- Do I believe the firmly rooted beliefs through which I view my life enlarge or block the flow of vital energy to my body?

- Do I believe that I'm here for a reason and that behind each challenge I encounter is an important lesson I am meant to learn? And, that if I don't "get" it, I'll keep "getting" it until I get it?

The idea that you actually experience what you focus your thoughts and feelings on is what this book is all about.

You have probably noticed that this book advances a few highly specific back-to-wellness factors and techniques. Central to the message is the notion that *you get in life what you focus your attention on*. But it may be difficult to maintain that focus unless mental images of illness are repeatedly replaced with optimistic pictures that serve a useful purpose. The result of this strategy of "replacement therapy" is a feeling of individual self-empowerment that can put you in greater charge of your life.

But to actually *succeed* in swinging our thoughts (and our health) in such a direction, repetition is the key. Each time you read a passage describing a key principle of wellness, the perspective and emphasis will be slightly different. The intent is to help you self-hypnotically register it in your memory and in your immune system response, so that you can eventually triumph over crisis. To prepare your mind for action, think of repetition as an enhancing force that sets off the Law of Attraction, giving you the immunity you desire from mental and physical illness.

Is the Law of Attraction at work this very minute?

Is it possible that you've been drawn, by expectation, strong desire, and feelings to read this material because you've unconsciously requested strategies to renew your mind, body and spirit? Read on and judge for yourself.

Chapter Two

Placebo: The Hidden "Miracle Maker" Within

The placebo is the doctor who resides within.
— Norman Cousins

In *The Psychobiology of Mind-Body Healing*, author Ernest Lawrence Rossi relates the story of a patient named Wright who had been diagnosed with lymphosarcoma, an advanced cancer of the lymph nodes. He also had very large tumors in his stomach, chest, neck, groin and armpit. His liver and spleen were enlarged. The condition was deemed to be incurable, and he was administered sedatives to comfort him in his waning days.

Wright himself was still hopeful he would recover, however. The reason for his optimism? He had read in the newspaper about a new medication for cancer called Krebiozen, and had also learned that the clinic at which his physician practiced was about to receive a supply of it to use in experimental tests. The rub was that only twelve patients were to receive the injection, and the tests were to be restricted to patients who were deemed to have at least three months to live. The doctors were convinced that Wright had only a few *days* to live. Wright, however, strongly *believed* that the drug would cure him, and he pleaded to be included in the study. To mollify him, the doctors agreed to include Wright in the study, figuring that once he had expired they would simply bring in a more promising patient.

To everyone's amazement, Wright had a profound transformation. A few days after receiving an injection of Krebiozen, he was walking around, the picture of health. In fact, of all the patients receiving a single injection of Krebiozen, he was the only one whose tumors had healed. Remarkable as it may seem, ten days later he was discharged from the hospital, and he was soon back to leading a normal life and even flying his airplane at twelve thousand feet with no uneasiness in breathing.

Within sixty days, however, reports began to appear in major newspapers highlighting the results of the study. The clinical trials suggested that Krebiozen was useless in the treatment of cancer. These reports had a most disquieting influence on Wright's mindset (and also his immune system). As negative clinical findings emerged in newspaper reports day after day, his spirits flagged. He felt more and more powerless to deal with his medical condition. As his expectation of getting well declined, his body's healing mechanisms weakened. After two months of almost perfect health, he deteriorated to his original condition.

When Wright's doctors saw the deterioration taking place, they leapt at the chance to double-check the sham drug, and perhaps determine how a patient's beliefs can, from time to time, bring on so-called "miracle" cures. Recognizing that a patient's unusual optimism may be a key to healing, they fed Wright an elaborate story about why the information he had read in the newspaper was false, and promised to administer an improved version of Krebiozen in a few days time.

Assured by his doctor that the new drug would work, Wright *expected* it to work—a powerful determinant in hastening the healing process. With all due dramatic flourish, the physician injected him a few days later with a placebo. His second restoration to health was even more startling than the first. Wright once again returned to health from a seemingly "insurmountable" illness.

Shortly thereafter, however, the American Medical Association came down hard on Krebiozen, announcing that "nationwide tests show Krebiozen to be a worthless drug in the treatment of cancer." Within forty-eight hours of this announcement, Wright entered the hospital in a terminal condition. Stripped of his images of hope, his immune response reduced its production of natural killer (NK) cells, so essential to ameliorating a life-threatening illness, and Wright passed away two days later.

Wright's case and countless others like it are examples of how placebos (harmless medications or medical procedures) prescribed by doctors can offer hope, and in so doing, can help unite a patient's body, mind, and spirit for a healthier life. Indeed, it is not uncommon for placebo pills to surpass those ascribed to a "real" drug. How can that be? It appears that the cumulative power of hetero-suggestion (belief transmitted from one individual to another)—can reframe maladaptive beliefs and optimize immune functioning (e.g., the production of natural killer (NK) cells.

An article published in the *New York Times* on January 9, 2000, titled, "The Placebo Prescription," delves into the placebo issue. The author, Margaret Talbot, brings to the table several scientific studies that have turned up thought-provoking results. In one study she mentions, ten military men requiring knee surgery were anesthetized. Of the ten, only two were given the operation that they were all expecting to undergo. The doctors merely rinsed the knee joints of three patients, and the other five weren't operated on at all. Instead, a little incision was made on the area to make it look as if the expected procedure had indeed been performed. None of the subjects knew which test group they were in, but six months later, all ten were pleased with their individual results.

Another study mentioned by Talbot involved an experimental technique for Parkinson's disease. Some of the subjects received the expected implants of fetal cells in the brain, other subjects did not. A hole was drilled to simulate the actual procedure in order to accurately test the placebo effect. Sure enough, the placebo group showed improvement, albeit not as markedly as those who actually received the implants.

The article also mentions the case of an allergy vaccine. Unfortunately for the British firm Peptide Therapeutics, its allergy vaccine proved to be no more effective than a placebo in controlled tests, and its stock fell 33 percent. Similarly, the pharmaceutical company Merck decided to stop developing a Prozac competitor it termed MK-869 when the placebo used in the study produced the same effect as the new drug. Genentech experienced similar results with a heart medication it was developing.

Irving Kirsch, a University of Connecticut psychologist, contends that antidepressants, Prozac for example, owe their success largely to the placebo effect. A study he conducted with Guy Saperstein from the Westwood Lodge in Massachusetts led him to the conclusion that a patient's belief in a drug is more powerful than any physiological change created by the drug. Kirsch asks, "Do people who are taking the drug do as well as people getting the placebo? The companies don't know and they don't want to know." Says Kirsch, "The critical factor is our beliefs about what's going to happen to us."

In yet another study discussed in Talbot's article, doctors cleared up warts for patients simply by brushing a bright dye made up of inactive ingredients on the area. The placebo effect also worked for conditions such as asthma. Subjects were told they were inhaling medication to open their bronchial tubes.

Dilation of the airways occurred even though they were inhaling a placebo.

The "real" issue!

Physicians need to spend more "high-touch" time commiserating with patients, many of whom are overly suggestible. This is a delicate undertaking, no doubt. Many doctors unwittingly distance themselves emotionally from patients. One reason is that under today's managed care programs—a high-tech, low-touch environment—the emphasis is on seeing more patients each day. Physicians, therefore, tend to spend less and less "high-touch" time communicating with patients. Even worse, some physicians become detached from their patients, not realizing that part of the healing process is to orchestrate patient perception (remember: there is no reality until it is perceived). This "distancing effect" reduces the likelihood that they will develop a therapeutic relationship with their patients. Practically speaking, in today's compressed patient-care environment, the physician really has little or no time to alter the mindset of patients who are often overwhelmed by negative emotions. Still, you wonder just how many doctors are aware that the energy lodged inside the emotion of fear, for example, can actually encourage chronic feelings of patient hopelessness, which in turn affects immune response.

The ideal situation, of course, is to have a "partnership" relationship with your doctor so you feel you have an ally in your struggle against a life-threatening illness. An empathetic doctor-patient relationship, in itself, can actually improve a patient's health, while the evidence suggests that many patients who *lack* an emotionally fulfilling relationship with their doctors can believe something serious is going on, and through negative self-suggestion and self-talk, can exacerbate or even bring on such a condition. A patient-imagined "worst-case" scenario can incite the subconscious into action, setting in operation the Law of Attraction. It should be remembered that:

A receptive mind attracts precisely what it expects (and worries most about).

Many physicians today believe that prescribing antibiotics for a viral condition is, in effect, prescribing a placebo, since antibiotics only treat bacterial conditions and not viruses. Yet the patients insist they need the drugs, and it is this belief alone that makes them seem to work. If thinking makes it so, you begin to wonder about the effects of vitamin supplements, and herbal and homeopathic remedies—particularly when they are suggested by a sensitive health care practitioner who is willing to extend the power of hope to stressed-out patients.

Physician attitude can actually influence patient brain waves yielding a sense of powerlessness or self-empowerment

All too often, physicians counter-intuitively suggest to patients, "Don't worry, I'll take over from here, trust me!" and other such rejoinders. As reasonable as these suggestions may sound, they can contribute heavily to patients resigning their power, thereby delegating it exclusively to the doctor and his or her technology. Such hetero-suggestions, if accepted, cause many patients to avoid taking responsibility of their own medical journey.

In most clinical settings such as doctor's offices and hospitals, patients are almost conditioned to expect bad news. A subtle relationship occurs between the physician (hypnotist) and the patient (subject), which can affect patient brain wave production. For example, if the association between doctor and patient is positive, relaxed, and empathetic, alpha brain wave activity will probably increase. Such brain-wave activity is associated with a state of relaxation, which enhances immune functioning.

On the other hand, if the physician is authoritarian and chilly, alpha brain wave activity is apt to decrease. If the doctor is detached and emotionless, the patient's increased anxiety can impair the immune system, which leads to further illness. In such situations, the patient gets precisely what he or she focuses on, which in this case are all-pervasive feelings of hopelessness and helplessness. Suggesting that patients turn their power and their emotions over to the doctor, thereby accepting a persona of powerlessness, can lead to pessimism. To better affect physiological functioning, patients should be encouraged to focus their mental images on thoughts of wellness, which will allow them to direct their behavior more pragmatically.

The problem, as I view it, is not with the doctor, but with the patient who allows his or her mind to become disempowered, and in so doing, blocks the body's defense mechanisms.

Checking your brain waves in a clinical setting

If one were to actually measure the brain waves (via an electroencephalograph or EEG machine) of people visiting physicians, I believe they would be distinctly different than those generated outside a medical environment. Patients in a clinical setting are almost egregiously conditioned to expect bad news. As a general rule, muscle tension increases and blood pressure is elevated. All of this presupposes higher-voltage brain-waves, as opposed to the slower alpha brain-waves associated with a state of relaxation, which combats stress and promotes the healing process. This is the reason why outcome-oriented visualization and the other mental programming exercises I describe in Appendix II are so important to use daily. Regular visualization practice allows you to enter a psychological alpha and alpha-theta state, which tends to positively alter the body's physiology. An even deeper state of relaxation is called theta, and deeper yet is delta. Many experts believe that bodily repair can be achieved in virtually any of these states.

Back in 1973, I experienced two watershed events that dramatically shaped my life. Number one, I became an assistant to a physician who was among the first to introduce biofeedback. As part of his research, the physician brought in the Swami Rama. The Swami had the ability to control his involuntary muscles, which science thought impossible. At will, he could alter the temperature of either hand by ten degrees, elevate his heart rate from 70 to 300 beats per minute, and, for a period of seventeen seconds, stop his heart with his mind. (As I recall, the original research was conducted at the Menninger Clinic, in Topeka, Kansas.) It was an astonishing demonstration of pure mind-body control—mental miracles might indeed be a more accurate description. And if that wasn't impressive enough, the Swami could, on command, generate alpha, theta and delta brain-waves. Beyond his disciplined control of his own body, the Swami had remarkable insight into the condition of others. A physician friend of mine witnessed numerous instances in which the Swami diagnosed ailments and dangerous events at a distance—one of which quite literally had saved my friend's life.

Similar diagnostic feats have been described by Jesse Sterns in *The Sleeping Prophet*. The subject of this book, Edgar Cayce, could diagnose and help treat illnesses at a distance, even while sleeping. In his wonderful book *The Edgar Cayce Remedies*, author

William A. GcGarey, MD, states that the famous intuitive "saw man as a traveler in time and space, a stranger on Earth, having his origin and his destiny in a spiritual realm, which we perceive most often only through the inner eyes and the words of those who have been given that privilege."

My second watershed event occurred back in the seventies when I signed up for an alpha mind control course. The course was designed to train students to invoke certain brain wave levels at will, in order to better manage weight problems, migraines, and other illnesses. We were taught to create an imaginary studio, where we visualized and acted out various outcomes we wanted to achieve on a mental screen surrounded by a white light. Before long we had created a imaginary movie with ourselves in the leading role, which we were instructed to replay religiously three times a day. Not surprisingly, the students who kept at it with expectations of positive results and the anticipation of adventure had uncommon success.

It didn't take attendees too long to realize that truly, in all of life, we alone are author, director and producer. Unfortunately, after about a year of practicing the techniques, I quit, not realizing that "if you don't use it, you lose it." I have since learned that in order to work effectively, the outcome-oriented visualization exercise has to become a part of your everyday consciousness.

Over the ages, Raja yoga masters and those like Swami Rama, have taken the practice of inner imagery even further, training themselves to move mentally from consciousness (the intellectual mind or beta state) to the subconscious (alpha-theta state), and finally to the superconscious, which encompasses the unity of all humankind and the universe at large.

It's my personal belief that people like Edgar Cayce, the Swami Rama, physician and medical intuitive Robert Jaffe, physician Judith Orloff (author of *Second Sight*), Dr. Carolyn Myss (author of *Anatomy of the Spirit*), and others are able to move mentally into an alpha-theta state because they are capable of tapping into the same vibratory frequency of their patients, hence their ability to identify specific realms of illness. I believe group prayer oscillation works much the same way.

A "wellness" coincidence

Recently, out of the blue, I received a call from a friend, who asked that I visit a physician diagnosed with inoperable cancer and conduct a mini-Quiet Miracles workshop. I contacted the physician's wife, also a medical doctor, and set up an appointment. I spent about two hours with the couple at their home during my visit, and left them with a great deal of information I use in my workshops.

About a week later, I was at the home of another physician, and during an idle moment my eye fell on a copy of *The Power of Alpha Thinking* by Jess Stern on his bookshelf. I asked my friend if I could borrow it. He said "Of course, even though quite honestly, I've never read it, nor do I know who gave it to me."

It was no accident that I felt so enriched reading the special book, a real energy-booster. It was like déjà vu. The book could easily have been my own autobiography. For example, Sterns described in detail the characteristics of autosuggestion, hypnosis, biofeedback, and the remarkable feats of Swami Rama. I had observed many of the same things firsthand while involved in biofeedback research during the same era.

The main subject of Stern's book, however, was a course in mind control that he'd taken which had enhanced his life significantly. I had taken the same exact course. He then went on to mention that noted physician Carl Simonton had taken the course as well, and it too had been a major influence on the invaluable health information presented to patients in his highly successful cancer center in Texas.

For the past five years, I had never given my own visualization technique a second thought. I assumed that I had created the technique. Not so. The main ingredients had been inspired by the course Stern was describing.

The next day, I asked the wife of the friend who had allowed me to borrow the book if I could lend it to the ill physician, since it blended in so seamlessly with the material I had left him and use in my workshops. She asked for his name. It turned out the ill physician and my friend's spouse were very good friends. Both couples being physicians, I supposed they had a great deal in common. To my no small surprise, she then pointed to a snapshot of the ill physician and his wife on one of the shelves in her home.

When I relayed this coincidence to the wife of the ill physician, her response was, "Isn't it a small world?" It is, indeed, but I hardly believe such "coincidences" are accidents. It's my firm belief that it's the old Law of Attraction in operation. And, if you have vivid confidence and expectation, it will work for you. It might be controversial, but that's how this creative "let's-make-it-happen" process works.

Prayer therapy

In the May 2000 issue of *HeartSense*, a knowledgeable monthly health publication by physician Stephen Sinatra (see **www.sinatramd.com**), he talks about the Apollo 13 mission and how, when disaster struck, people from all over the country prayed for the safe landing of the mission crew members. It's his personal belief that the nation's collective prayers may have been instrumental in saving their lives.

In 1988, studies conducted by Dr. R.C. Byrd of California and other researchers, added support to the notion that intercessory prayer can beneficially affect patients' medical conditions. Byrd tested prayer as a means to improve recovery rates of patients. He chose three hundred ninety-three patients who were in critical care and split them into two groups. One group was treated with standard methods. The other group unknowingly had people outside the hospital praying for them.

Byrd's results were so profound that nine researchers sought to duplicate his findings. More than a thousand patients were used in the follow-up study. The researchers determined that prayer could help traditional medicine in healing patients. The participants did not all have the same religious beliefs. A belief in God was a common bond among the patients.

Physician Larry Dossey, in his book *Healing Words*, cites a number of reputable studies that bear out Byrd's results in regard to the benefits of prayer "intervention." Dr. Dossey muses that, had the prayer intervention been a drug, people would have been clamoring to know precisely what it was! The researchers summarized their findings by stating that "prayer may be an effective adjunct to standard medical care." Still, the subject is controversial and some recent studies have cast doubt on the idea that prayer is good medicine.

Looking for help in all the wrong places

In looking for help outside of themselves, rather than to the "healer within," patients are more apt to radically delay the healing process. It's natural to worry and to be afraid. However, instead of looking at the toxic beliefs within us to resolve emotional issues, we look outside for answers. Fear shakes us all up, so we do everything we can to avoid it. Consequently, there is little time away from the emotion, nor do we make time to set the issue aside and come up with a solution. Fear and the failure to face the reason for our fear drains energy we need to remap and heal ourselves. Consequently, the same stressful drama gets played in our head over and over again. Being smack in the middle of fear, we have trouble even convincing ourselves we can deal with it. The moment we choose to move out of the flight stage and mentally envision stepping in and facing the emotion, we stop being frightened.

It helps to ask yourself, "What could I be learning from this fearful life experience?" The answer could be found by taking action to resolve it, moving forward through and beyond it. Obviously, this requires self-discipline and a meaningful shift in thinking. It means being mindful of the importance of taking control rather than being controlled by a medical condition or life circumstance.

Be assured that once you experience the re-energizing feeling of taking charge of your own destiny, you will stop burning up precious energy needlessly. Taking a pro-active part in facing fear, uncensored by negative beliefs, will help you do just that. But you've got to realize it's not only the medical community that incites your mind to envision fearful images—it's you. The solution is to be your own gatekeeper and the leading spokesperson for yourself, which means taking full responsibility for your own medical journey. To maintain that feeling of self-empowerment, you must remain actively involved in seeking out the best of conventional and complementary care, while at the same time leaving the reactions of past self-destructive beliefs behind you once and for all and moving forward to a healthier mental state.

Some physicians naturally dispense placebos, which can accelerate the healing process.

Many doctors dispense placebos as a matter of course, by their very manner, which gives their patients greater opportunities to overcome illness and improve their quality of life. Empathetic and sensitive, these doctors—walking placebos—are well-equipped to help those highly suggestive patients who often get themselves unduly worked-up. In effect, these physicians are powerful immune system stimulators. Through the power of direct suggestion and soft, gentle, reassuring touch, they empower patients by altering their toxic beliefs and assuring them that they can trigger their *own* inner resources to heal themselves. It seems rather obvious that a doctor's personal influence can heighten a patient's confidence and thereby encourage better health. Such a physician becomes an instrument for setting the mental actions essential to healing into motion.

The doctor can encourage patients to activate their own body defenses against disease, yet . . .

Each patient must fully cooperate in the back-to-wellness process by adding heightened intensity and emotional intent to reinforce mental images of wellness. Self-initiation in dealing directly with self-limiting beliefs and thoughts is a critical component in the wellness equation. Without full awareness of your existing self-destructive beliefs and expectations, it's far too easy to fall back on entrenched thoughts of helplessness and hopelessness.

Michael Crichton, a Harvard-trained physician and author of *Jurassic Park*, *The Andromeda Strain*, and other best-sellers, writes in his book, *Travels*, that it's important to keep the purpose of the physician in perspective. "The doctor," says Crichton, "is not a miracle worker who can magically save us but, rather, an expert adviser who can assist you in your own recovery."

The only expectations you have to meet are your own.

Only by taking responsibility for your own thoughts and feelings can you move forward toward recovery. Interviews with long-term cancer survivors underscore this key fact—in order to recover you must seize control of your mental imagery on a daily basis. You must form constructive beliefs and thoughts, using Infinite Energy as the shaper of life experiences you envision and strongly desire. By continually expanding your mind's boundaries through the practice of outcome-oriented visualization and the wellness exercises detailed in Appendix II, you will be thinking your way to solving daily challenges far more effectively than ever before.

Chapter Three

Do You Make These Mistakes in Sabotaging Your Health?

If we all did what we are capable of,
we would astound ourselves.

– Thomas Edison

Ten years ago, a friend decided to have a personal color chart study taken to determine the best colors to wear based on her complexion, hair, anatomy, lunar cycle, and other assorted information. One day, while looking for a swimsuit, she spotted a garment that looked particularly becoming. In fact, it had her name written all over it. But alas, it didn't fall within the color-scheme that had become a "given" in her life. She had become convinced that certain shades were "definitely not right for her," and decided not to purchase the item. To this day, she automatically rejects any color that does not appear on the pallette she has devised for herself. And perhaps she will never discard or override the highly suggestive beliefs (rules) that she artificially created and brought into existence—ten years ago.

The "real" symptoms of illness.

Imagine now what happens when an individual who is completely convinced there's no imaginable way they can restore their health, (a) creates highly suggestive mental imagery that focuses intently on symptoms (which often they have memorized) said to be attributable to the illness, (b) which leads to even more pessimistic pictures of the illness, (c) which reinforces the existing condition.

If you're completely convinced (via self- or hetero-suggestion) that you'll remain ill, this is precisely what you will continue to attract and bring into your life experience. People tend to identify with their established beliefs which "The Law of Attraction" fosters and brings into physical existence. An unchanging belief about what's possible and what's impossible intensely colors your world. Perhaps Abraham Lincoln summed it up best when he said that "people are about as happy as they make up their minds to be."

How to alter your undermining beliefs!

To alter a framework of damaging moods, begin by asking yourself if the firm beliefs that underly and reflect your disposition are life-enriching. Do they translate to feelings of wellness? If your answer is no, reject and replace them using the "Suspension of Damaging Techniques" strategy in Appendix II.

To get a better handle on how your negative beliefs bring about negative life conditions, ask yourself the following question: "*What circumstances am I attracting into my life through the power of my toxic beliefs and thoughts?*" Make it a point each day to examine the corrosive beliefs you're focusing on, reinforcing, and actualizing, perhaps almost subconsciously. This is a particularly tough regimen to follow, because it's easier to dwell on forces seemingly beyond your control that have brought about your condition. The answer to the question, "What life experiences am I attracting into my life?" requires that patients take full ownership for the circumstances in their life, which overturns everything they have learned. Yet this is the perspective of many long-term cancer survivors. It's one reason that these individuals have been able to transcend medical statistics, reinventing the world as they envision it.

Catastrophic beliefs can be discarded through the healing energy of outcome-oriented visualization and the other strategies detailed in Appendix II, if you are willing to confront and silence them. Keep in mind that by reducing your self-destructive beliefs, you lift your spirits, harness wellness energy, and become your own instrument of wellness.

"Freedom," said Robert Frost, "lies in being bold."

How many hours a day do you spend worrying? By boldly examining and altering adverse beliefs that delay healing, you'll soon become aware that the same energy you waste generating feelings of pessimism can be directed toward implementing a wellness action plan. If you remain skeptical that you have the latent ability to generate bodily health and draw into your life beneficial life experiences, tell yourself:

> *It could well be that if I make up my mind to move beyond my self-destructive thoughts and feelings, choosing wellness over despair, I'll create healthier options and realizations. This is going to take a major investment on my part—a willingness to work on elevating my "Toxic Belief Awareness Index"—a truthful assessment of the negative beliefs, thoughts, and feelings that my mind seems to switch on daily.*

The Helen Keller/Nike advertisement "Just Do It!" Strategy. (*Really* Do It!)

You can rid yourself of fear and despair if you learn to focus your attention on your *strengths*, not your weaknesses. As I mentioned earlier, Helen Keller, though deaf, blind, and bereft of speech at nineteen months of age, nevertheless lifted herself to a high level of attainment by using her remaining abilities to move from the role of victim to that of victor. You can achieve similar results through the dedicated practice of outcome-oriented visualization, autosuggestion, positive self-talk and the other wellness exercises revealed in later chapters. Being a victor means visualizing yourself as a victor. It means moving from thoughts of "I'll give outcome-oriented imagery and the other wellness strategies a try," to "I'll *really* do it and make them work!" There's a vast difference between these two actions. Embracing one or the other can quite frankly lead you to success or failure.

Once the Law of Attraction begins to take hold through the motivating force of positive belief and repeated mental imagery, beneficial results are virtually assured. It's been my experience that many cures deemed incurable by the scientific community are the result of the power of belief, which formidably sets the Law of Attraction to work at a subconscious and biological level.

When a picture (mental image) is worth more than 1,000 words!

It's important to remind yourself repeatedly that your body is the physical materialization of your mental images and emotions, which are powerful forms of creative energy. They have energetic impetus. Focus on improving your mental images and your body will repair itself. Seeing the mental image you want to achieve as already completed attracts to you its attainment. "What lies behind us and what lies before us are tiny matters compared to what lies within us," said Ralph Waldo Emerson. Your mental images bring experience into your life and they serve to reproduce themselves outwardly following the doctrine: "As within, so without."

Your mental images generate virtually all psychological and emotional issues in your life. Contaminated mental images, which give rise to destructive emotions, can sabotage your body's defense system by blocking healing energy, thereby causing physical deterioration. Squander your vital energy on negative beliefs—a physical violation—and the alienating effect on your immune system is highly likely.

Crisis can be a great teacher!

Crisis can awaken self-destructive beliefs residing within you, or it can be a great teacher, helping you to move forward on your personal journey. It can remind you that indeed, you are a spiritual being connected to Infinite Energy, a limitless power within that can assist you in radically enriching your physical and mental well-being. To find the doorway to better health and accelerate healing, however, it is important that you consciously rid yourself of toxic mental images and thoughts. Better health demands that you remain ever aware that daily, your mental images (which reflect your central beliefs and thoughts) shape your private inner and outer world.

When was the last time that you held your dark thoughts and feelings up to the light of day? Learning how to identify, examine, and manipulate the images of your beliefs, thoughts, expectations, and feelings is what earth's classroom is meant to teach you. One thing is certain: Life is not a spectator sport. You must be a participant in order to rise above your self-sabotaging beliefs and thoughts. Such beliefs are your own personal version of reality, be it of wellness or illness. Your imagination is a drafting board. With continued commitment, use it to design vivid mental images of wellness. One long-term cancer survivor put it this way: If you believe you'll heal or if you believe you won't, from your point of view, you're absolutely right.

To transform your life—it is critical you learn to displace your debilitating links to illness.

To reverse illness, there are specific universal laws to which you must fully awaken. Physician and medical intuitive Robert Jaffe states that a *direct link* exists between the damaging belief imagery that you focus on (hypnotize yourself to believe) and daily reinforce—such as the debilitating energy of past hurts, blames, anger, resentment, not forgiving someone, fault-finding and jealousy—and the *blockage of healing energy*. Unless you undue your toxic beliefs, they can attract and create dysfunctional conditions (e.g., a sense of powerlessness) and disease states to enter your life. Out of control, they will continue to do their damage until you choose to take action to remedy them.

The body expresses what the mind perceives. What you perceive, you experience.

Most people fail to realize that much like interest on an old loan, disease-causing pessimistic mental images and toxic feelings compound daily. The psychological emotions you convey through your sabotaging beliefs and thoughts affect your entire biological makeup and physical experience. Having the courage and attitude of mind to understand this synergy will help you change your disruptive beliefs.

Chapter Four

Startling Facts
About Miracles

I first came across the material described below when a doctor friend suggested I obtain an audiotape of Dr. Bruce Lipton, a former medical school professor at Harvard and at the University of Wisconsin's School of Medicine. He is the author of *The Biology of Belief*.

Dr. Lipton discusses a Harvard geneticist and biochemist named Dr. John Cairns who, in 1988, published in *Scientific American* what he believes to be the most important paper in the history of biology. Dr. Cairns denies the notion of random cellular mutation as put forth by Charles Darwin, who proposed the idea that elements of heredity are passed on from parent to offspring. Some have also claimed that psychological traits are transmitted from parents to offspring. Conversely, Dr. Cairns said specific genetic alterations are brought on by environmental conditions. His contention: the environment, rather than genetics, is the determining factor in cellular mutation.

Dr. Cairns' findings came while working with bacteria that were unable to process lactose. The bacteria were lactose intolerant and had no enzyme to break down and digest the lactose sugar molecules. He placed the bacteria in Petri dishes in which the only nourishment available was lactose. Dr. Cairns did this believing the bacteria would be greatly stressed, since they would be unable to nourish and sustain themselves. They were not expected to reproduce in the Petri dish, since they did not possess an enzyme to break down the lactose. Yet robust colonies of bacteria developed in all the Petri dishes. How?

Dr. Cairns found that the bacteria, provided with an inadequate source of nourishment, adjusted their digestive elements to adapt to the food source.

They adapted to the environment by altering their genes in order to create an enzyme that could digest lactose, a mechanism now known as adaptive mutation.

What Cairns discovered was this:

Organisms have the inherent ability to alter their genetics to adapt to the environment.

This means that genes do not transform by pure chance, as Darwinism had suggested. Rather, genes change by intent in order to adjust and make full use of their environment.

No matter what antigen or foreign substance is introduced into the body, cells have the capacity to create a gene that will produce a neutralizing product—which is called an antibody (a blood protein that counters an antigen). The cell produces an antibody in response to each stress it encounters in the environment. That is to say, when an organism encounters stress, it can modify (mutate) its genes to accommodate the stress. This is not, as Darwin proposed, an accident or a random event.

Also, cells do not change all of their genes in response to environmental signals. They tend to alter very specific groups of genes that are directly related to the stress. This is called adaptive mutation and takes randomness out of the equation of life. What this tells us is that organisms, by their very nature, are able to adjust to the environment they find themselves in. Therefore, it is not DNA that controls us. It is the environment and our response to the environment that can turn DNA on or off in our genes.

Dr. Lipton suggests that it is our interpretation of the environment that selects the DNA that makes up the genes. In other words, we have in our cellular characteristics, genes that can adapt to the environment by intelligently rewriting genetic code. Contrary to what was previously thought,

The nucleus of the cell (which contains the genes) is NOT the brains but simply a computer disk containing all of the cell's architectural plans.

It might be helpful to consider the analogy of a home computer. If you remove a disk from a computer and hold it in your hand it cannot execute a function. The reason: The disk merely holds information. It has long been believed that genes (which, like a computer disk, hold information) also have the ability to turn programs on and off. Lipton's experiements suggest that genes cannot switch themselves on and off, any more than computer discs can. They are merely reproductive structures. When cells break down, genes contain the plans to reproduce them as required. But genes do not control cell life. A gene is a chemical that is incapable of turning itself on or off. It is simply a blueprint; a magnetic tape that holds information.

But if this is so, then what *does* turn a gene on and off? Dr. Lipton believes that the switch is in the cell membrane which contains receptor proteins. Each of the receptors has antennae embedded in it that interface with the external environment.

What this tells us, says Dr. Lipton is this:

**Organisms do not evolve by a random process—
without conscious choice—but in a manner that
is directed by consciousness.**

It bears repeating that it is now recognized that there are specific genes called genetic engineering genes whose sole function is to rewrite existing genes in order to accommodate the environment. It is now known, says Dr. Lipton, that—

**ANTENNAS on cell membranes represent
the true brain of the cell (much like a computer chip),
while the nucleus of the cell (which contains the
genes) is merely the disk where
the processing takes place.**

Dr. Lipton maintains that genes are no more than blueprints composed of DNA and these units of heredity are altered as required by environmental demands. The key to recognize, he says, is that genes do not govern our biology. Rather it is our perception of the environment that strongly influences our physical structure, behavior, and gene activity. He makes that statement because

**Receptors represent our awareness of the
environment through the medium of the physical
senses, which, by definition, is perception.**

The big "AHA" is this: Genes do not control your cells; perception or belief—your personal interpretation of the environment—is what controls your cells.

Genes can be changed by your beliefs.

Stated yet another way,

You get what you focus on!

Your *focus* determines the information that's available to your genes. You can exercise your innate power to alter your life by changing your belief-focus, your desires and your intents. Genetic determinism is not inherent in our structure, says Dr. Lipton. Again, we are NOT victims of heredity.

The key element for change is *perception*!
(focused beliefs, thoughts and expectations).

We are controlled by perception. This is in line with what Quantum physics is suggesting: Namely, *there is no reality until it is perceived reality*. If, for example, you're under extreme stress, you almost automatically alter your biology (physiology). What Dr. Lipton is stating is this:

Your beliefs, thoughts and emotions are your biology!
They limit or expand your world.

Dr. Barbara McClintock discovered that genes rewrite themselves on a daily basis to accommodate our perception of the environment. She won a Nobel Prize for her work (though recognition was very slow in coming). What Dr. McClintock proved is that *cells are programmable*, and as quickly as you can think a new thought, you activate body mechanisms that program the expression of your cells. Dr. Lipton says that this accounts for such states as multiple personality disorder (MPD) and the placebo effect. He

says this is why MPD patients experience such dramatic physiological alteration when they undergo a deep psychological change.
Amazingly, their bodies respond physically, often in seconds. This
demonstrates that *cells are programmable* and, as you program in
new data, your cells accommodate the data.

Nature is Intelligent.

Sadly, says Dr. Lipton, Darwinian biology to a considerable
extent hypnotized people into focusing on feelings of hopelessness, helplessness, and general powerlessness. Many people
believe they are simply "gene machines;" their fate has been
decided in advance and they cannot influence or mold it. Living
in this kind of toxic mindset, people come to believe they are
powerless victims of some genetic history. Becoming aware that
consciousness has other modes of perceiving information is critical to becoming well.

What is finally being realized is that

Organisms can energetically
rewrite their inherited genetic messages.

Of prime importance, says Dr. Lipton, is that quantum physics
combined with cellular biology is now able to take note of sub-
cellular actions. The big reveal is that

Your beliefs can actually rewrite your genes.

In those terms, if you change your beliefs, you can alter your life.
You are more powerful than you ever imagined. You are not helpless. You are only a victim of your beliefs, which you can willfully alter. Beliefs mold and influence your future. They are the

rules you live by. So any belief, thought or expectation, spoken or thought, implies an action, an expression.

Psychologists maintain that seventy percent of our beliefs are negative in nature. Since every cell is listening to your every thought (energy in motion), it's easy to see that your positive or negative beliefs, thoughts and expectations can, in physical terms, not only affect your behavior, but the functioning of your immune system as well.

Before quantum physics, science mistakenly believed the nucleus was the command center or brain of the cell because this is where the genes are located.

It's now recognized that the function of the cell's nucleus is to engineer programs and blueprints, and to replace parts for reproduction. The genome project has demonstrated that, if you remove the nucleus of a cell, the cell continues to function. Also, if you remove the genes, the cell will continue to function. However, if you remove the antennas on the receptors of the cell's membrane, everything shuts down. Hence, the brain of the cell is the membrane, which has receptors (proteins) with antennas.

Our gene programs are not set for life.

Biologists now recognize that genes are susceptible to alterations. In the language of science, genes are subject to mutations or change. In Darwinian Theory, the concept of "random mutations" implies that evolution of life on this planet is purely the result of chance. This is wedded to the idea that all of life resulted by accidents (random mutations) with absolutely no intent or purpose underlying it.

Francis Crick, who discovered DNA, advanced a similarly fatalistic theory. Unfortunately, this view is so widely held that some women with a history of breast cancer in their families have undergone a total mastectomy rather than risk contracting it. Dr. Lipton says that a belief that you will be diagnosed with cancer is a perception that promotes the development of cancer. This points to the fact that you cannot separate your beliefs from your biology.

Dr. Lipton says that less than seven percent of breast cancer or other illnesses are genetic in origin. This means that ninety-three percent of breast cancer has no genetic linkage. Scientists are now slowly beginning to recognize that through our perceptions and our beliefs, we relay information to our body that can reorganize our immune system. We thus generate our own illness or wellness.

Self-limiting beliefs, the placebo effect, and the discouraging impact of biological theories that fail to acknowledge the active role of the mind in shaping personal health, are all, in one way or another, aspects of the phenomenon I'm describing. Still another example is:

Multiple Personality Disorder (MPD)

How is it that people with multiple personality disorder (MPD) can demonstrate a number of organic conditions —each materializing a *distinct immune response*—depending on which personality is being acted out?

In my book, *Quiet Miracles*, I write about an "acting-as-if" phenomenon that I found characteristic of long-term cancer patients that applies to the MPD subject at hand. Let me quote the book:

61

To be added to medicine's growing bank of knowledge is a striking phenomenon that proves the mind-body connection very strongly—and shows that the acting-as-if concept has a legitimate medical explanation. As mentioned earlier, studies have shown that patients who have multiple personality disorder (MPD) can, depending on which personality is present, demonstrate different bodily characteristics, including dermatologic reactions, seizure disorders, and allergies.

In the *American Journal of Clinical Hypnosis* (Volume 26, No. 2, Oct. 1983) an article entitled "Psychophysiology Phenomena in Multiple Personality and Hypnosis," Bennett G. Braun, M.D., describes neurophysiologic differences between MPD patients and control groups. In his study, all but one of a patient's personalities were allergic to citrus juices. When the host personality (the one who has control of the physical body) ate an orange, no ill effects occurred. However, if another personality took control too soon after the orange was eaten, a rash would develop.

In another example, a female MPD patient had one personality who was extremely allergic to cat dander. When this personality was exposed to a cat, the patient would experience a runny nose and eyes, wheezing, and a rash. However, when another personality was in control, she could play with a cat for a time without any allergic reaction.

Dr. Braun discussed many such cases of MPD, all equally surprising. Clearly, such cases reveal the existence of a profound mind-body connection. The conclusion is clear: If MPD patients can experience actual physical differences (acting literally as if a separate personality is present), then all human beings share the capacity to alter their physical condition with their mind.

Like Dr. Braun, Dale Anderson M.D., the author of *Act Now!* has described several MPD examples and another even more revealing study that shows how to dramatically enhance your immune system function and improve your health. Dr. Anderson cited the study conducted by Nicolas Hall and Maureen O'Grady, professors of psychiatry and behavioral medicine at the University of South Florida, and Denis Calandra, chairman of the department of theater at the same university. Their report was published in *Advances: The Journal of Mind-Body Health*. These researchers drew a sample of a MPD patient's blood when each personality was present. At one point, they took a blood sample within seconds of the time between the end of one personality's appearance and the start of a subsequent one. They found a large variance between the personalities and their immune responses. In other words,

**Each transformation of personality produced a
different chemical profile
merely because of the way they thought about disease.**

The researcher's conclusion:

**We become as we act.
"Act As If" you are healthy and your
physiology improves.**

To confirm that patients with MPD have multiple immune systems, Professor Hall studied two members of the University of South Florida's theater department. The actors were given two plays—a comedy and a depressing drama—to perform. For several weeks blood samples were taken from the actors at many points during rehearsals and performances. Comparisons of the results of the blood analysis revealed that there is indeed a correlation between personality and the immune system response. Simply put, these actors proved that when you are feeling or

"*Acting As If*" you're happy and optimistic, your body chemistry is different from that when you're feeling sad or pessimistic. Professor Hall noted "Results like these are less surprising when we remember something about the nature of emotion: *Feelings are chemicals, and chemicals are feelings.*"

**The point is that "*Acting As If*" can become real!
Your body cannot tell the difference.**

I have certainly experienced this truth in my own life. I have had blue moments, times of sorrow, periods of darkness when I believed things would turn out badly. They seemed endless, although they really only lasted for a few days. Each period felt like a term of imprisonment, and it was at these times that I gave thought to giving up the battle. My carving of despair was my own creation, my choice, and I ignored anything that did not seem to fit my filtered belief. Just as an actor reacts negatively while playing a depressing role, so too did my body react to my gloomy attitude. I felt lousy.

The obvious dawned on me one day after rereading Victor E. Frankl's book, *Man's Search for Meaning* and finding the operative quote:

> *Everything can be taken from a man but one thing: the last of the human freedoms—to choose one's attitude in any given set of circumstances, to choose one's own way.*

As I focused on that mind-altering phrase, I told myself that (a) I alone had the power to choose each moment as a new healing opportunity, (b) I was free to effectively reject cancer and deal with its attending fear component, and (c) "acting as if" I was okay was the pathway to healing I would choose.

A Major "Aha."

In adopting contaminating beliefs, thoughts and feelings through focused mental imagery and self-suggestion (generally due to chaotic stress and strong fear), MPD patients act *as if* they are distinct personalities. Within the context of their existence, this action generates dramatic chemical changes in their body, causing biological alterations in their immune response. A major "Aha": Each immune response that emanates from the presence of a distinct personality is a reflection of the interior images and thoughts it focuses on. The significant lesson that can open you to securing wellness is:

Your body expresses what your mind perceives.

Clearly, the body's immune system is geared to, and biologically altered by, the emotional focus of whichever personality emerges. The different interpretation (perception) of each MPD personality, which emanates first from the imagination's subjective reality, forms feelings which influence changes in the body's defense system. Can you now see that your inner world of beliefs and thoughts gives rise to your physical experience? Understanding that feelings are chemicals, and chemicals are feelings—inner dimensions that give rise to your state of affairs—suggests that you have the inherent power to choose your subjective world which forms your daily bodily existence.

Here is the wellness delivery system you can learn from those with MPD:

- Modify your inner world through your inherent ability to change your toxic mental imagery and feelings.

- Use positive self-talk (messages you continually send to yourself) to nullify past and present emotional hurts.

- Act as if your new perspective or belief is already achieved.

As art imitates life, how you interpret a given situation creates your physical existence. Since each thought is embedded physiologically in every cell of your body, why not start implanting new, powerful self-healing beliefs in your imagination this very minute?

**You become your beliefs, thoughts and feelings.
Think and feel it and...it will come!**

Let's summarize the central premise that your individual interpretation of events color your beliefs which, in turn, strive for physical realization. Generally, MPD patients imaginatively focus their attention on creating new beliefs to escape disturbing emotional circumstances, such as tortuous sexual abuse. Science is now coming to believe that MPD patients learn to adroitly play radically new life roles—an undertaking which they unconsciously believe is essential to transcending the chaotic infractions of their life.

Ever faithful to the spirit of the transformative roles they act out (attributable to the imaginative new belief structures they've constructed and ardently focus upon), MPD patients are unaware that the performance of each personality sets in motion the Law of Attraction, which fosters change in their entire mental and physical makeup.

Do the physical occurrences experienced by MPD patients correspond to how cancer survivors beat their life-threatening illnesss, against all odds? I think they do.

Learning to throw the "wellness belief switch."

Taking the conclusons of the MPD research to their logical extreme, it would seem feasible that you could create an emotionally sanitized version of MPD in patients with life-threatening illnesses, teaching them how to throw a "wellness belief switch," so that a new, healthy immune system would emerge. This may seem like a speculative, far-fetched notion, but all of us, in one way or another, are play-acting this same scenario each day of our lives, as our moods and aspirations shape our vision of reality, and also our sense of opportunities and disappointments.

The biochemical and vibrational influence of bad feeling thoughts on your health and life experiences.

By now you can begin to see the principles in action when people, in response to their emotional outlook, act as if they already are victims. In feeling both hopeless and helpless, they attract more of the same experiences back into their lives. This is why it is so critical to override toxic thoughts and recreate yourself with planned purpose.

Do you ever feel pushed to the edge?

When you're sorrowful and pessimistic, your body chemistry is different than when you're happy and optimistic. Certainly, when you're immersed in a state of self-suggestive powerlessness, hopelessness and helplessness, the disease-promoting energy of this condition manifests itself in every cell and vital organ of your body—making it virtually impossible for you to gain control over the back-to-wellness process. The focus and intensity of your beliefs and feelings activate (or deactivate) the body's biochemical healing processes, which can thereby attract either constructive or destructive life circumstances to you. The Buddha captured this illuminating dharma (key Buddhist truth) when he said, *"The mind is everything; what you think you become."*

Chapter Five

Straight Talk About
Well-meaning but
Toxic Conversations.

Watching yourself getting hooked into toxic beliefs of illness demonstrates how the victim lying dormant within
you can quickly become activated. Understandably, when a person
first learns of his or her chronic illness or is faced with a crisis, he
or she often feels victimized. It is easy to paint negative mental
pictures and get derailed emotionally when a crisis takes place. It
is also easy to understand why all of us want someone to lean on
and nurture us through distress—someone to support our way
of thinking—someone sympathetic to reinforce our personal
plight. "But watch out," says Dr. Carolyn Myss, author of *Why
People Don't Heal*, "because there seems to be an unwritten belief
among many people, that, to connect with others—a basic human
need—we have to intimately share our feelings of victimhood.
The problem: Bad feeling thoughts, talked about and focused on,
vibrationally attract and form matching future experiences!

Have you ever noticed how some people can subtly hook you
into self-pity, almost without your knowing? These people seem
to revel in the victim mentality, forgetting or perhaps unaware
that negative thoughts have pulsating energy—a biochemical
force that can damage the body by attracting more of that same

negativity into your life. Such exchanges of despair can suck the energy right out of your immune system. One of my physician friends refers to this as "psychic vampirism."

Watch out for the "Voice of Victimhood"!

When "victims" send their negative attitude and messages in your direction, it's important that you go within to interrupt and disperse these intense feelings. If you don't, they're likely to join forces with your own deeply rooted destructive beliefs. The gap between the highly rational mentality of the long-term cancer survivor and that of the emotionally charged victim is never more pronounced than when victims repeatedly chronicle their travails.

It's clear that a toxic mindset can be contagious and can break down the body's immune response. Therefore, looking to connect with people by swapping weaknesses (e.g. gloom, depression, sadness, misfortune, sorrow) seldom contributes to well-being. As you listen to other people exchange calamities, it will become clear how emotionally toxic such conversations can be—not unlike a powerful television broadcast. Those who focus on and transmit despair send self-sabotaging messages not only to themselves, but to others who have "tuned in" to the same frequency. What's really taking place is an *amplifying input–output exchange of live, destructive emotional energy, which can reduce the utility of the body's defense system and attract further debilitating events into your life.*

Just the facts, please!

Here's an example of how toxic thought-transmission works: In one of my workshops, a highly despairing young woman described her chronic illness and began to lament the painful blows that life was dealing to her. Like a deadly contagious disease killing the flow of all positive energy in its path, her injurious thoughts and harmful feelings, even though well-intentioned, spread rapidly through the workshop affecting virtually every attendee. Her bleak disposition and continued despair incited the image-forming power of all who were receptive to her (and their own) hopelessness, and quickened the flow of negative energy through the mental domains of each emotionally involved attendee, leaving many of them fully hypnotized into feelings of self-pity, which caused physical occurrences to take firm hold during that session.

It is understandable that those who are living in a world of pain will look to connect with kindred spirits. Unfortunately, such sympathies generate corrosive thought-energy of such sympathies—think of it as a victim emotional virus—in those who receive them. The hookup and interaction can take place with binary speed, not unlike "spam" e-mail targeted digitally from one in-box to another.

What's going on is a kind of *quid pro quo* energy drain that you want to avert at all costs.

This poisonous exchange of feeling is something you definitely want to shun. You might want to think of it as a software virus that can infect and weaken your entire bodily structure. When someone wants to exchange woes, be mindful that what takes place is not unlike a hypnotist-subject relationship, where the subject accepts the belief of the hypnotist.

I later wrote a play about the occurrence I've just described, which I sometimes use in workshops as a role-playing device. The incident vividly demonstrated how the shift in thought and emotions can take place so quickly and deeply that the resulting physical and emotional harm is initially invisible. The irony is that five therapists attending the session could do little or nothing to stop the negative suggestions received and the functional disturbances they caused to those with receptive minds. Like nearly everyone else in the room, I found *myself* vulnerable, emotionally smothered and hooked firmly into the contaminating energy of victim despair. The effect was so powerful, in fact, that I removed the exercise from subsequent workshops. On the contrary, the *Quiet Miracles* workshops are now based on creating a feel-good place by means of the Law of Intended Consequences.

The message, the whole message and nothing but the message!

That workshop experience taught me the vast creative power of mental imagery and feeling, which incites the mind to secure the results on which you focus your thoughts—either favorable or unfavorable. The clear message:

All of us get what we intensely center our mental focus upon.
Again, what you think and feel, you become!

From that day forward, I knew with absolute certainty that never again would I play host to such a mental and physical violation without quickly challenging it. Attendees are sometimes taken aback, in fact, by my abrupt response to their toxic mental focus and verbal exchanges. What they initially fail to "get" is the higher realization that: (a) mental imagery of strength can gain victory over thoughts of weakness, and (b) one can put an immediate halt to an exchange of harmful, vibrating energy by summoning forth hopeful and optimistic inner images and self-talk (autosuggestion)—a power possessed by virtually everyone. The early detection system I now use to exterminate potentially toxic exchanges in my workshops is to (a) stop and quickly point out the inhibiting emotions being emitted that are offering an alternate view of reality, (b) quickly ask the attendee involved what corrective belief-reorientation action he or she plans to take to disconnect from his or her psychological and emotional trauma(s), and (c) ask the attendee to draw meaning from the experience, thereby advancing his or her own spiritual development. It's interesting to note that most toxic energy exchanges are initiated by attendees who have made little effort to practice the survival tools detailed in the workshop (and in this book).

Every thought and feeling attempts to become real!

You need to recognize that morbid beliefs and thoughts are *powerful forms of transforming energy* that can easily impact every aspect of your life. You'll be reminded throughout this book that your body believes every word you think and responds in like fashion. In order to maintain your total health emotionally and physically, you must become aware of how the transference of negative beliefs and thoughts can anchor and manifest themselves in your mind and body.

How to be your own gatekeeper and the leading spokesperson for yourself.

Have no part of an exchange in hopelessness and helplessness, or the attending fearful feeling it generates. If you do open the door to fear, then through the *Law of Attraction* (like attracts like), you'll materialize precisely what you fear most. Engaging in sustained talk and feelings about your illness with others creates a thoroughly negative atmosphere and mindset, which is hardly the way to promote health and tranquility. On occasion, I have to remind attendees that,

The purpose of the workshop is growth in self-empowerment, not growth in powerlessness.

The objective of my *Quiet Miracles* workshops is to remind people that they already possess the power within to break out of the mold of negativity. The *Daily Wellness Action Plan* provided at the end of this book, if assiduously practiced, is the key to healing on all planes—emotional, physical and spiritual.

To effectively shield yourself from an epidemic of toxic mental imagery and emotions, the best plan is to put yourself in a conquering mental state, thus preventing crippling thoughts from targeting, occupying, and becoming a fixed habit of mind. Unless you take control of circumstances, circumstances will control you. In confronting toxic energy exchanges, you will be forced to face and challenge your own as well as other people's self-defeating hopelessness. For my part, it is a matter of helping workshop attendees who are willing to help themselves out of an intractable emotional exchange.

Someone once said that there is no easy road to learning. It took me years of workshop experience to learn that true self-empowerment, growth and transformation can be achieved naturally by mastering your mental images, by believing you can attain the outcome you intensely envision and holding to it until it becomes "fact."

Does this mean you should avoid discussing emotional issues with others? Not entirely. But you need to follow up such interactions with positive, *self-empowering* action. You must encourage people to challenge the beliefs that engender their feelings of powerlessness. As I have so often witnessed in my workshops, assisting attendees to reframe their negative beliefs triggers a flow of energetic well-being, which effectively attracts healing to them. The resultant atmosphere of infectious good spirits can relieve stress, generate hope, and set optimism (a true catalyst to healing) astir.

Bonding in the wrong way!

Sometimes it seems that we can only get close to one another by sharing our painful wounds. We may believe we are tapping into someone else's source of strength, failing to understand that this paralyzing exchange can block the flow of energy to the body's vital organs. And by entering into another's contaminating thoughts and feelings, we reinforce our own as well. There is great truth in the expression "misery loves company." For this reason, I make it a special point to be in the company of people who naturally "accentuate the positive and eliminate the negative." It is not an easy matter but, whenever possible, I try consciously to create a controlled therapeutic inner and outer environment. (Note: See Appendix II for the major weapons at your command.)

Do you ever examine the lens through which you see life? Look closely, it'll give you a living picture of yourself and a Preview of Coming Atractions!

Sadly, there are some patients who blame their physician for their illness and the notion that they're unable to speedily get well. They insist on receiving certain drugs and operations they may not necessarily need, while simply refusing to take charge of their own medical journey and life. When the doctor can no longer help them, they blame everyone but themselves for their condition. They feel powerless to change their medical condition, and come to believe that they will inevitably succumb to it. Anchored in negative beliefs and feelings of discouragement, they truly believe they do not have the ability to self-suggestively place themselves in a mental state that can alter their ill health. This intense emotional state paralyzes the very images they need to summons in order to live a positive life. The lens of illness through which they view life colors their perception of the outer world.

Medical statistics: another case of anchoring one's belief in powerlessness.

It is not an exaggeration to say that the emphasis on death statistics is yet another illness-promoting mechanism that can contribute to sustained images of powerlessness and its severe side effects. Therefore, it's well worth reminding ourselves that

Statistics do NOT apply to individuals!

Give this some thought: What percentage of the people who are diagnosed with a life-threatening illness dedicate themselves to the essential strategies prescribed in this book? Is it even one percent? Now ask yourself this: "Of this one percent who focuses their abilities on wellness, what percentage do you believe have turned around a chronic illness? It's a number, I believe, that's far greater than statistics now being published.

There is truly an element of the irrational in any approach that can mass induce an unfavorable mental state in the public's psyche. For example: When was the last time you heard a statistic like, "89 percent of the population is safe from a heart attack?" Is it conceivable that actuarial statistics are self-fulfilling? Is it possible, too, that those with highly receptive minds and those that choose to accept negative statistical data imaginatively magnify their own conditions and bring about that statistic?

How often do we hear someone pessimistically remark, "My mom died of cancer when she was in her early sixties; it'll probably be the same for me. You know, statistics say that kind of thing runs in families." Ever thought about the power of self-suggestion summoned into the mind and fully at work in that telling statement? It might well be that, through fearful self-suggestion, people who accept the harmful belief that they have no power over their mind and body effectively define their own potential. After all, if you magnify your self-limitations, you erect your own mental prisons. The result: You can't outperform your own self-definition. The magic belief to absorb is this: *"There are no limits for journeys of the mind."*

Are today's public advertisements of prescription drugs a help or a hindrance?

Whenever you develop stress about your condition, do you say to yourself, "I can either take pill 'X', or I can take the time to practice outcome-oriented visualization in order to resolve the tough emotional issues behind my condition?" It seems pretty obvious that subsisting on pills alone, without therapy, merely strengthens the powerless belief that you're "stressed out." By choosing to continue your medication without resolving the emotional issue behind the stress, you fail to perceive your mental state affects your body—that they are indeed, "one." If you continue to take pills for anxiety (which the media regularly advises us to do), you may lose your incentive to identify and resolve the psychological or emotional issue that lies at the heart of your stress.

Are the health successes claimed for vitamin supplements, herbal products, aromatherapy, healing pendants, and the like, a form of auto-suggestion?

The authors of advertising copy are well aware that claims such as "This vitamin or herb will cure you of such and such a disease," and "Wearing this pendant will get you that which you most desire," can often sway the mind, bringing about precisely the results attributed to the medication or treatment. They fully understand that expectation, in the form of descriptive mental pictures, is a major element preparing a receptive mind for the suggestions given.

Drug-drug and drug-food interactions.

Is it likely that highly suggestive patients who familiarize themselves with the possible adverse side effects of prescription drugs influence their own immune responses. This being the case, you can see how it happens that when such people are alerted to a drug side effects, they form and reinforce matching effects in their bodies. And what about foods that yesterday's news told you were dangerous to your health, yet today are nutritious? We're told that certain foods contain pesticides which are poisonous to our system, while others can establish a healthier condition. What mental imagery are we creating for ourselves by following these suggestions which change almost daily? It's far better to direct the power of your mind to suggestions that offer feelings of self-empowerment and hopefulness. By practicing the Wellness Action Plan suggested in a later chapter you will be able to ward off dangerous foods and toxins, clean up your internal as well as your external environment, construct a healthy condition of mind and body, and nullify the adverse environment around you. Along the way your entire mindset will be brightened.

In short, what you *expect*, you get.

Ever notice your state of mind when you watch a gifted magician at work? No matter how mystifying the performance, deep down, you know each event has a rational explanation. I once saw The Great Blackstone perform a seemingly miraculous event. His show opened with a search light pointed to a woman locked into a cage high above the audience. Suddenly the room darkened. In a matter of a second, the search light showed the woman in the cage appearing on the stage next to Blackstone. How was this masterful illusion achieved? I had to scratch my head in wonder. Still, the audience got what they expected. The intent of the magician was to precondition the audience by placing it into a receptive state of mind, in order to make the illusions "real." This is similar to ads that condition our minds to believe a given message by repeating it *ad nauseum*. (Incidentally, the "cage trick" was accomplished using identical twins.)

Unlike a magician's performance, events are not circumstances that merely happen "out of the blue." They are actualized conditions formed by you according to your beliefs and emotions. You see evidence of this in people who expect the very worst to happen—and it usually does. These are people who say, "Well, at my age and in my condition, everything is downhill from here." But in a sense, you can understand where they're coming from. Today, unless you have your wellness sensors up, you have no idea what treatment option or set of clinical studies to believe, since they so often contradict and repudiate one another. And once the media *interprets* the findings, confusion becomes the order of the day. Here is something else to think about: Having been associated with scientists who are on the payroll of large corporations conducting studies, I have to wonder if the results are credible and in the best interest of patient welfare—or in the best interest of those paying for the research?

A reasonable suggestion to advertising agencies and their giant clients

The mind has a powerful intuitive defense system that can immunize itself to bring about a state of health and well-being. Why not put its natural immunity to work by inoculating the American public with suggestive mental images emphasizing the body's natural power to heal itself? Why not have real physicians speak confidently about the positive belief and feelings used by survivors to beat life-threatening illnesses!

Rather than health announcements and ads which mirror people's fears, the American public could be sent repeated imagery that cancer, for instance, is not always fatal. Physicians could point out the great truth behind the principle of focusing on positive and powerful outcome-based mental imagery. By receiving these "messages of wellness," the American public would begin to develop greater confidence and trust in the picture-forming power of their minds.

You don't have to take it anymore. Here's the combination for unlocking your own power for wellness:

1. Don't ever allow yourself to wallow in self-pity and be led astray by harmful hetero-suggestive statements, either

public or private, that keep toxic victim-energy locked inside, thus delaying your health and well-being.

2. Encourage yourself (and others) to grow emotionally and spiritually stronger rather than allowing yourself to lock into someone else's past hurts. "Bonding" in this manner only blocks energy needed for wellness on all levels of your being.

3. Look closely at your unresolved emotional issues and find the cause behind them. Be aware that either you control the emotional energy blocked within you, or it controls you. For example, if you're going through a difficult divorce, the toxic energy of anger can quite literally induce the malfunctioning of your immune system, which, according to the *Law of Attraction, draws to you more of the same.* Until you quit empowering what's behind your anger, such as unfinished divorce issues, you will not experience health and well-being no matter how strongly you desire it. Forgiving others and yourself has enormous immune-enriching power.

4. Remind yourself of the advice physician Dale Anderson offers in his book "*Act Now*": If you *act as if* you're going to get well and you act with confidence, your body's physiology will change and you can begin to create the way you act, thus empowering your immune system.

5. Unplug from the toxic energy of a chronic illness and address even the most challenging situations by reassessing your values and asking yourself: "*What essential life lesson is this crisis meant to teach me?*" Choose to look

at crisis as a rare opportunity for further self-discovery leading to higher planes of consciousness.

6. Understand that, in all of life, you attract to yourself the circumstances on which you intensely concentrate.

Daily, life is full of important feel-good or feel-bad choices—the consequences of which no one can avoid.

Damaging beliefs, yours and others, are easier to identify than you think. If you examine your current life experiences, closely, you may note difficulties you have attracted to yourself by your lamentations and expectations. Look for the harmful, self-destructive beliefs, thoughts, and feelings hidden behind them. Start putting your priorities in place by re-evaluating the life choices that contribute to your laments and the life conditions you have formed. For example, ask yourself, "Do I often relate to others by sharing past and present wounds?" "Do I dwell on images of illness, thereby indulging in victim consciousness?" "Am I constantly talking about my illness?" Again, be aware that this is blocked energy that you need to release in order to reverse chronic conditions.

Understand that if you repeatedly hook people into your sorrows, you can harm them. Instead, act as a poster person for supreme optimism and joy.

Make it a special point to conquer negativity by bringing a happy face and a cheerful attitude to your encounters with other people via the "Acting As If" Principle. If they choose to lock in to your cheerfulness their immune system will function better for having been in your presence. Make it a daily practice to select healthier beliefs and you'll notice your focus of attention changing from negative to positive, and that will go a long way to tipping your immune functioning scale to the side of wellness.

Envision and FEEL yourself triumphing over adversity

Believe deeply that you have the inner power to alter your mental energy field. Say to yourself, "Every day in every way, I AM getting healthier and healthier. Through my energized thoughts I can realize the outcome I strongly desire." Now visualize and feel your goal, e.g. "see" wellness, as physical "fact."

Are you *really* prepared to accelerate your back-to-wellness potential? Ask yourself these questions to find out.

- Do I *really* want to change my dominant negative thoughts and feelings?

- Deep down, do I really believe that I experience what I focus attention on?

- Can I actually picture myself identifying and countering my self-destructive thoughts and feelings?

- Do I honestly believe it's possible to visualize the outcome I strongly desire as *already* achieved?

- Will I practice a results-oriented visualization exercise often enough (three times a day) and long enough (30 days), to give it an opportunity to take hold?

- Do I realize that I'll experience the precise amount of

difficulty altering my thoughts and feelings that I expect to meet?

- Am I willing to take the time and effort to write down my core beliefs on a piece of paper and closely examine them?

- Am I willing to take the time and effort *daily* to write down the experiences I want to enter my life, knowing inwardly that by my focus, I can actualize my thoughts and feelings into physical reality?

- Do I believe that I'll continue to attract to myself negative emotions and influences unless and until I take it into my own hands to identify and resolve them?

- Do I understand that relentlessly practicing outcome-oriented visualization and other back-to-wellness techniques are absolutes for success?

- Is procrastination and inertia a reality in my life?

Beating procrastination by mastering the art of relentless persistence.

If you answered "yes" to the above questions, you'll understand Dr. Norman Vincent Peale's advice in his famous book *The Power of Positive Thinking* that "nobody in life ever won a victory over anything without persistence and perseverance." In his writings, he quotes inspirational luminaries such as Göethe, who said, "Austere perseverance, harsh and continuous ... rarely fails its purpose, for its silent power grows irresistibly greater with time." Dr. Peale also quotes Shakespeare who offered this sage advice, "Much rain wears the marble." Still, the quote I feel carries the most significance is by Burke, who said, "Never despair; but if you do, work on despair." Remember now: you create only the life you perceive—what you focus energy on.

Caution:

In my opinion, it takes more than the power of positive thinking to rid yourself of negative events that enter your life. You must actively examine your self-destructive beliefs and feelings and replace them with positive, higher frequency, feeling-good thoughts with persistent intention and strong emotion. In this way you'll attract similarly positive events into your daily life. The fact that you have been attracted to this book is a good sign, and it's no accident. As you continue on with it, you will learn how, by the strength of relentless persistence, you can overturn a framework of self-destructive beliefs and replace it with one of possibilities you imagine as already achieved. Such an opportunity is readily available to virtually anyone willing to boldly explore their inner being. What's required is a sustained belief that you can take the "t" out of can't, and a willingness as a *conscious co-creator* to actually *do it*. Unless we face this challenge—unless we digest the cosmic lessons this lifetime is meant to teach us, and align ourselves with Divine Energy—we will be held back in life's classroom that our soul signed up for.

Chapter 6

Thousands Can Make a Miracle – But Never Learn How. Meet the "Barrier-breakers."

Do you happen to recall the name Roger Bannister? He was the British fellow who in 1954 was the first to run one mile in under four minutes. Until he broke the four-minute mile barrier, the mindset of all runners was that this was a "mission impossible." At the time, Bannister's accomplishment was called the "Miracle of the Century."

Of course, you've heard of Helen Keller. At nineteen months, acute congestion left her deaf, blind, and mute. Yet later, she graduated from Radcliffe College, winning the school's highest scholastic honors.

If you think about it, these "mission impossible" stories are not about breaking the four-minute mile or other physical barriers.

**These stories are about
"breaking the mental-barrier"—
about making the so-called "impossible" possible!**

What's most revealing about these and other barrier-breaking experiences is that they offer one simple truth that all of us should incorporate into our lives: You can't outperform your own self-definition—your self-limiting thoughts, beliefs, expectations and feelings!

Here's why I make that statement: Once people like Bannister and Keller broke the seemingly insurmountable barriers in their particular fields, others quickly came along and broke them too. The barrier was largely a mental one, in other words, knowing that it *could* be done made these so-called "impossible" tasks suddenly far easier to accomplish.

These stories teach us a formidable lesson about the creative power that belief gives us to meet challenges. The lesson is two-fold: It's only our narrow perceptions that limit us and,

The *boundaries* or *limits* we mentally set for ourselves are nothing more than *imaginary* lines.

The imaginary lines that defined the boundaries for runners and also for those with physical limitations were mental constructs that withered as soon as someone demonstrated that they were not iron-clad.

Okay, why do I tell you all these stories?

Well, as I mentioned, back in 1995, I was diagnosed with cancer. As a practical guy, faced with the possibility of dying, I began to examine my options in life: (a) I could work myself into hysterical panic, (b) I could put my head under the covers, or (c) I could take control of my medical journey and my life. The real question was: Would I take full charge of my medical journey or wouldn't I?

To begin with, I needed to learn how to empower myself, and quickly. I searched wide and deep for specific information on how long-term survivors beat cancer. I read what Bernie Siegal, Carl Simonton, Andrew Weil, Depak Chopra, Joan

Borysenko and others advised. Frankly, the information was quite overwhelming.

At the time, I remember reading an article about Willie Sutton. He was the famous bank robber, who when asked, "Why do you rob banks?" responded by saying "Because that's where the money is!" Following similar lines, I decided to begin interviewing long-term cancer survivors, many of whom had been diagnosed as "incurable" by the scientific community. After almost three years of research, it became obvious to me that not all cancer patients die—even if they have a seemingly "terminal" condition. Somehow, these ordinary people more than occasionally accomplish an extraordinary feat: they break the healing barrier.

Naturally, I wanted to pick the brains of these survivors for the secrets to their success. I wanted to make those secrets work for me. I wanted to know the rules by which healing success is attained. And sure enough, I began to observe key characteristics that long-term cancer patients had in common.

But before I tell you about the specifics of my personal journey, let me tell you a bit about my background. I've been a student of altered states of consciousness since my days at University of Minnesota High School. For a brief period while subsequently attending the University of Minnesota, I was a research assistant in hypnosis experiments in the psychology department. As mentioned earlier, I had also been involved in biofeedback experiments witnessing Swami Rama (whose case study had been detailed by the Menninger Clinic) perform some rather amazing physical feats using nothing more than his mind. For example, he could control his involuntary muscles. I also have a degree in pharmacy from the University of Minnesota. For many years I was the Chairman and CEO of Pharmacy Corporation of America, a public company.

With my scientific background, you might guess that my workshops stress a medical approach to wellness. That's true. I tell attendees that I believe one should freely choose the best of allopathic and complementary therapeutic alternatives—making certain that at all times they allow their physician to monitor their progress.

So now that you have a sense of my background, let me tell you about my own remarkable experiences. When I was diagnosed with cancer, I constructed an "outcome-oriented visualization" technique (picturing the outcome I wanted to achieve as already accomplished) called a "mental healing temple." This was based on my knowledge of auto-suggestion, meditation, and other complementary healing modalities.

Initially, I considered myself to be the world's worst visualizer, and that, of course, was precisely what I experienced. As a result, most often I only *heard* the narrative I was trying to create, rather than actually *seeing* it. Yet one day, in attempting to construct a mental healing temple, my deceased mother remarkably appeared, cupping the area of my face where the cancer had been detected. It was a highly emotional moment and I included that mental imagery in all of my subsequent visualizations sessions, which I practiced intensely three times a day—when I awoke, when I was tired and just before dozing off—the times when we are most susceptible to suggestion and least resistant to outside distractions.

Then, on August 9, 1995, something quite extraordinary happened. I had been incorporating several of the long-term survival techniques (described in detail in Appendix II), along with unhooking from a negative focus and instead choosing good-feeling beliefs to focus on. That evening, in the middle of my nightly visualization practice, I felt a firm hand—that of my dead mother—slowly cover the right side of my face, the exact area where the malignant tumor had been diagnosed. At first, I thought my wife had touched my face. Not so. The "hand" remained for approximately one minute.

The next day, after my normal workout on a NordicTrack® exercise machine, I decided to lie peacefully on the floor and rest for a few moments. Two or three minutes later, I felt two gentle "hands" cupping my face. Startled, I stiffened. For a split second I thought someone was standing over me and had placed both their hands on my face. I opened my eyes. I was alone. My breath stopped. Nevertheless, I made the decision to "go with it." About three minutes later, I could feel an indescribable power outage take place and the pressure of the cupped hands lightened and vanished. When I arose from the floor, I placed my hands on the area the "hands" had touched. I could no longer feel the tumor on the right side of my face.

On my next visit to my oncologist, I mentioned this incident. Understandably, my doctor said he would do his own "physical." Finally, after 15 minutes of examination, he said, "You pass."

Now unless you have experienced a consciousness-altering or paranormal event first hand—and I've had several—it is very easy to doubt their existence. Nor do you know the limits of your own inner capabilities unless you have seriously attempted to use visual imagery and the other tools described herein to stretch your subjective boundaries.

It's always astonishing to me that many people know so little about the fundamentals of outcome-oriented visualization—envisioning the result you want to achieve as already accomplished. Yet I believe it's an essential catalyst for accelerating health and well-being. This strategy should be one of the highest priorities in any back-to-wellness process. The reason: Such an intensely combative mind-clearing approach tends to wipe away negative beliefs and thoughts in virtually all aspects of your life. By sharing what I've learned, I hope to help others learn the fundamentals of outcome- or results-oriented visualization.

Let William L. Fischer, author of *How to Fight Cancer and Win*, explain to you the power of visual imagery therapy:

> *At age four-and-a-half, Sara was brought in to see Leslie Salov, M.D, the former director of the Vision and Health Center in Whitewater Wisconsin. Suffering from blood tumors behind her left eyeball, Sara's eyesight was growing worse with quick progression, to the point where it was evident the eyeball would have to be removed along with the tumor.*
>
> *Dr. Salov explained in simple language to Sara exactly what the medical problem was, and began to teach her a visual imagery technique that he himself had used when his eyesight began failing from a degenerative condition. Within eleven months with continued visual imagery, Sara's vision was virtually back to normal.*
>
> *Being an M.D., you might wonder how Salov became interested in visual imagery. Nothing to lose and quite desperate, he decided to try visualization therapy. Initially, he was quite doubting since he thought it was out of the sphere of medical science. Eventually though, he became a strong supporter of visual imagery. But that was only after Dr. Salov gained back 75 percent of his eyesight.*

Clearly, such cases reveal the existence of a profound mind-body connection. I also believe if multiple personality disorder (MPD) patients can literally hypnotize themselves into experiencing actual physical differences (acting literally "as if" a separate personality is present which automatically alters their immune response), then all of us share the capacity to dramatically alter our physical condition by acting as if we can.

Here's still another piece of the wellness puzzle to examine.

A study was conducted by Nicholas Hall and Maureen O'Grady, professors of psychiatry and behavioral medicine at the University of South Florida, along with D. Calandra, chairman of the department of theater at the University.

Professor Nicholas Hall studied two groups of the University of South Florida's theater department. The actors were given two plays—a comedy and a depressing drama to perform. For several weeks blood samples were taken from the actors at many points during rehearsals and performances. Comparisons of the results of the blood analysis revealed that there is indeed a correlation between personality and the immune system response. Simply stated, these actors proved that when you're feeling or "Acting As If" you're happy and optimistic, your body chemistry is far different from that when you're feeling sad, stressed out or just plain pessimistic. Professor Hall noted this: "Results like these are less surprising when we remember something about the nature of emotion: *Feelings are chemicals, and chemicals are feelings. The key: You become as you act.*

In the *Quiet Miracles* workshops I conduct, we discuss precisely how negative emotions send damaging chemical messages to the physical body. Here's the explanation: Catecholamines, which are neurotransmitters (hormones that send messages from cell to cell), become reduced when you're in a negative emotional state. As a result of the catecholamine action, your endorphin levels increase as well. The outcome: Your immune system reduces its functioning.

With this information available to them, workshop attendees become aware of how negative self-talk—a terribly destructive form of self-hypnosis—directly affects their immune system and blocks the healing process. The lesson: *"Acting As If" can become real! Your body can't tell the difference.*

A deep understanding of the above studies coupled with safe, simple, and effective exercises can help people voluntarily deal with their damaging thoughts. I believe this vital information can offer virtually anyone with a chronic illness the essential tools necessary to fight it. This does require, however, opening yourself to new information, plus the courage to risk taking control of your own well-being. I often tell attendees of my workshops that the one thing I definitely cannot provide them with is the inner will to RISK stretching their self-limiting mental boundaries so they can empower themselves to move forward with their life. *Indeed, batteries are not included in my* Quiet Miracles *workshop. The inner summons must come from you.*

My belief is that taking risks and breaking barriers is what life is all about. Repeatedly, long-term cancer survivors voiced this invaluable advice: To be a "barrier breaker," you must take charge of our own medical journey—and your life—and you should take this freedom very, very seriously.

I've discovered that many people who've survived a life-threatening illness have awakened to the realization that, in order to persevere, it's essential they be their own gatekeeper. They've learned, often the hard way, to speak up on their own behalf. Even under the most difficult circumstances, they've learned the importance of being the leading spokesperson for themselves. It's emotionally self-empowering, and it activates all of the body's inner workings.

We cannot become what we need to be by remaining what we are.

– Philosopher Max Depree

For the most part, in the case of long-term cancer survivors, it's clear that what we are dealing with are "barrier breakers" with an active willingness and intent to open new life frontiers by:

- consciously changing their toxic beliefs, thoughts and feelings and setting new goals and purposes,
- practicing outcome-oriented visualization,
- facing and releasing the toxic affects of psycho-emotional issues that block healing, and
- daily rehearsing success via the "Acting As If" strategy.

Here's another interesting thing I've observed: When you ask people why they believe they contracted a life-threatening illness, they will tell you they understand the reasons fully. They tell you they had an acrimonious marriage, a failed personal relationship, a highly stressful job that "was killing me," a spouse that was an alcoholic, and so forth. Their belief is that a constant build-up of toxic psychological and emotional uncertainties and adverse conditions brought on their illness.

As a result of the relationship between virulent psycho-emotional issues and illness, I encourage people under highly stressful conditions to seek professional advice immediately. By taking such action, they are wisely choosing to take control of their medical journey and life problems, though it may require a 180-degree shift in their negative beliefs—what Zen masters sometimes call moving to the "witness state" (e.g., distancing yourself from your highly suggestive beliefs and thoughts).

Energetic healing.

In my judgment, barrier-breaking requires learning more about how the body's energy fields regulate well-being and how to begin to work with those energies to restore your health. This is not as cutting edge as it sounds. Sub-atomic physicists now talk about an energy field that exists everywhere, which they refer to as the "near surround."

Are you a victim of the beliefs, thoughts and feelings you hold?

One thing to become ever more aware of is that disbelief—closing your mind to life's ever-expanding healing options—severely limits your potential for healing, self-understanding, self-empowerment and spiritual growth. For my part, I try very hard to keep my mental receptor sites open to information that can stretch my mind and my healing options. On the stage of life, I would rather be sorry for *what I tried* than for *what I did not try*. Reverend Martin Roloff conveyed this notion when he stated, "The giraffe feeds where others can't reach." That's my philosophy: To aim for things we think we cannot reach." Winston Churchill, expressed it this way: "You shape your dwelling, and then afterward, your dwelling shapes you."

By expanding your boundaries and breaking mental barriers, you make it possible for something quite extraordinary and profound to happen. The potential is almost always there.

Meet physician and "imaginary boundary-breaker" Elisabeth Kubler Ross, M.D.

Perhaps some of the pieces to life's puzzle transcend conventional thought. Maybe, just maybe, there are other dimensions of reality that we're missing because our mental receptor sites are closed. For example, during my search to gain further spiritual growth, I attended a small, spellbinding meeting at which physician Elisabeth Kubler-Ross was the guest speaker. You may recall that she is the author of numerous books, her most famous being, *On Death and Dying*. She also originated the concept of hospices.

One of the many extraordinary stories Dr. Kubler-Ross told us that eventful evening may give you a true sense of her personal discoveries. She noted that one day, one of her little patients must have sensed very clearly that she was about to leave this life. The doctor said she saw evidence of this in the child's statements and conduct. Then, several hours later, the young patient approached the doctor and said, "Doctor Ross, I 'see' my mother and father on the other side, reaching out for me."

Dr. Kubler-Ross explained to the child that she had called her parents and at that very instant they were motoring by car from their out-of-state home. She asked the child to please wait for her parents to arrive. The youngster failed to cooperate and passed away. Later that day, Dr. Ross learned that while driving to be at their daughter's side, both parents had been killed in a car accident. Dr. Kubler-Ross explained this phenomenon as follows: "When you die, it's not the end of your journey. It's the beginning of a totally different existence. All you do when you die is just drop your physical body like a cocoon, then a butterfly comes out of it. Your soul continues to live through endless existences, literally."

Let me tell you still another of my favorite barrier-breaking stories. It is the reason why one of my personal life philosophies is …

"Leap and the net will appear."

It is the story of the kindergarten teacher who asks her little student, "Sally, what are you drawing a picture of?"

"I'm drawing a picture of God," responded the child.

"But sweetheart, nobody knows what God looks like," said the teacher.

"They will in a minute," said the little student.

The child responded as she did because children begin with the unrealizable, which is the point where most adults often stop.

Although the barrier-breaking material outlined here has had a profound impact on my own life, I advise workshop attendees not to simply take my word for it. Rather, I encourage them to make a deliberate effort to uncover these important life experiences themselves. It is only by making such a mental "shift-in-consciousness" that they will begin to activate the energy needed to gain the results they desire.

Breaking barriers means going within to get unstuck from old emotional "issues."

In the end, all of us must uncover life's major truths for ourselves. During my healing journey I've learned that the answers we're all looking for are within, not without. Again, what's within gives birth to what's without. Therefore, the best strategy to change life's "externals" is to change your internal mindscape. The lesson is that to change the course of an illness, or any existing negative circumstance for that matter, you need to stay in charge of your beliefs, thoughts and feelings, rather than replaying the old tired dramas. Could it be that this is the primary lesson we all need to learn in order to allow our highest destinies to surface?

Chapter 7

"Medical Intuitives" (Physicians) Who Practice Tomorrow's Next Big Scientific Cures Today!

Does the term "medical intuitives" leave you feeling uneasy, if not downright skeptical? Before you judge what I'm writing as quackery, marketing hype, or New Age mysticism, I implore you to read on. Then close your eyes, take a deep breath, and momentarily "turn off" the analytical left side of your brain.

That's exactly what I had to do. I'm by nature analytical and scientific. I'm also deeply spiritual. And I had cancer. In my desire to reconcile my two sometimes conflicting ways of looking at life and heal myself, I discovered how to integrate conventional and complementary medicine, and it has brought a powerful new force into my life, which I want to share with you.

Intuitives.

Some gifted people are able to transcend the limitations of the five senses and "read" the distinct energetic frequencies that govern the physical, emotional and spiritual functions of the physical body—the Chakras. In some cultures such people are venerated, while in others, such as our own, they are often scorned. But whatever their title and status, one point deserves emphasis:

these intuitives, no matter which culture they come from, agree on both the appearance and interdependency of the energy patterns to which they are uniquely attuned. They also agree that electromagnetic dissonance in any of the major energy centers (or Chakras) can indicate potential disease.

The nourishing energy fields emanating from the Chakras are called *etheric* energies. They are described by medical intuitives as invisible streams of vitality indispensable to life. They form the harmonic link between the physical, emotional, and mental aspects of each human being. If there is an uninterrupted flow of this subtle, nutritive life energy, good health in the organ systems of the body can be maintained. But if this vital flow of life energy becomes blocked because of inner emotional imbalance or dysfunction, it can undermine a person's health.

Intuitives can see the auras (different frequencies of energy) around someone's Chakras change with that individual's changing health. Any significant change in the body's subtle energy field is immediately evident in the Chakras. For example, a healthy person will demonstrate symmetrical Chakra energy patterns and exhibit a distinctive "rhythm", which is moving in an integrated harmonic pattern.

If that person becomes ill or upset, the aura, or band of energy surrounding him or her, will appear to be darkened. Intuitives can see a multicolored aura of moving anger vibrations (intense concentrations of emotional energy) manifest itself in a highly energized solar plexus Chakra where these strong vibrations clothe themselves. Such inner anger (which can cause immune system suppression) can be seen by distinguishing the shading, position and color of the energy patterns that accompany an emotional charge.

An excellent book on this topic is *The Chakras and the Human Energy Fields* by Shafica Karagulla, M.D., a neuropsychiatrist, and Dora van Gelder Kunz, an exceptional clairvoyant blessed with the ability to perceive not only the body's etheric (vital) field and its major life energy centers (Chakras), but also the integrated higher astral (emotional) and mental fields with their corresponding interactive energy centers. The authors' empirical research indicates that an individual who's happy will display a specific pink pattern energy frequency and a person who is in meditation or prayer will exhibit a vibrational overlay of blue and gold.

A gifted intuitive can "see" imbalance and blockage of vital energy flow.

According to Karagulla and Kunz, there's a constant interaction not only among the three energy fields (mental, emotional and spiritual), but also between these fields and fields of vibration operating at a higher and perhaps universal level. A practiced intuitive can transfer and help regulate vital life energy flow between this multi-dimensional universal field and the organs of the physical body. This relationship between personal Chakras and a larger energy field makes it possible to reverse abnormalities and restore balance to a dysfunctional Chakra, though it will entail treating the *whole* person rather than using the more conventional approach of treating the physical body as a structure of unconnected parts. An intuitive "sees" the mind, body and spirit as inseparable, and treats them as such.

For centuries, Eastern doctors and intuitives have shown that abnormalities observed in one or more of the specific energy centers are indicative of a tendency toward disease.

Medical intuitives have noted the relationship between a non-working Chakra's energy pattern and physical symptoms, and that with early detection of these abnormalities, severe diseases can be predicted *prior to the body's manifestation of the physical symptoms.* They've also shown that what appears to originate in one energy level may actually derive from a deeper source, such as the emotional or mental state which can cause immune deficiencies in the body. A tumor, for example, may appear to originate at the solar plexus, yet its luminous and rapidly moving energy discharge may derive from a deeper emotional level of consciousness, such as unresolved stress or anger. Unresolved stress or anger reduces the flow of vital energy and inhibits the normal functioning of an organ system in the body. Contrast this with a happy and harmonious inner frame of mind, which is mirrored in the Chakras as a healthy flow of higher vibrational nutritive energies, which can affect permanent physical body healing by enhancing mental and spiritual well-being.

The interaction of the seven Chakras is a continuous process, and changes in the subtle energy exchanges, or alterations of rhythm in these centers of energy, and are what cause weakness or maintain bodily well-being. This is why knowledge of the Chakras can be both a diagnostic and a therapeutic tool—Chakras are the energy sites at which great healing can occur.

A number of well-respected medical doctors and intuitives, no longer limited to Eastern philosophy, live and practice in the United States today.

Be aware, however, that there are countless charlatans in the world who offer "sure-fire," "get-well-quick," "miracle" cures. It is right to be skeptical in these matters. However, do not let these false claiming individuals deter you from finding *gifted* medical intuitives.

One trusted practitioner is Robert Jaffe, MD. Jaffe is both a medical doctor and an experienced medical intuitive who has already helped countless patients by clairvoyantly seeing disease before it physically manifests in the body. He believes, as do many others who are attuned to human energy fields, that we're all multidimensional creatures. In his view our soul exists as a higher vibrational state, just as our physical body is a lower state and our emotional body is an intermediate aspect of our being. These differing aspects are intimately connected in subtle ways through a network of energy channels to form the cellular structure of each individual—a structure that regulates and maintains health.

As strange as this may sound to some, Jaffe says that he can often look inside a person's complex energy network, discover what's out of vibrational balance, predict the energetic consequence, and alter the energy flow to restore that balance. For example, when faced with a patient who has a thyroid condition, he "sees" that there is a dense, dark blue energy in the thyroid that has affected body physiology. Since this Chakra or energy center area often has to do with the dynamics of self-expression, he takes under consideration the fact that the patient has difficulty expressing him or herself. By asking pointed questions, he may discover this to be true. He then tries to find the underlying reason behind this abnormality. For example, what happened in the patient's past that influenced this dysfunction? The next step is to guide the patient to face the root of the illness and thereby resolve the conflict. If the patient is receptive to the idea that they indeed are sending negative energy to themselves, Jaffee claims he can actually observe the subtle vibrational energy in the thyroid untwist itself.

Like many intuitives, Jaffe believes that permanent healing can not occur until we handle the psycho-emotional aspects behind our disease.

Clearly, then, the healing process is much more complicated than just taking a pill or undergoing an operation. Instead of curing the underlying cause of many problems, therefore, modern physicians often merely postpone the inevitable. For instance, if a person is suffering from heart disease and the arteries are opened, the condition is temporarily fixed, but the underlying emotional problem has not necessarily been resolved.

While part of the solution may be diet and medication, Jaffe believes physicians should look deeper into the effect that a patient's psychological processes may have on his or her biological system. Subconscious or half-acknowledged beliefs or thoughts can suppress the immune system, and for this reason, the mind's influence on the body must be addressed if a cure is to be found.

Jaffe offers an example of the biochemical influence of emotion upon health. While traditional medical doctors are uncertain of what causes kidney stones to develop, Jaffe believes they are the result of tension and currents of fear (unresolved trauma, anger, resentment, etc.) that are held in the kidney area. These predisposing factors can cause a contraction of the energy field (Chakra blockage), which increasingly affects the biochemistry of the body. Eventually, a kidney stone will develop. If, however, he can convince the patient to address the root cause underlying the symptoms, which can move the powerful energy currents of fear out of the Chakra area, balance is restored and the stone can be prevented.

Jaffe has also had several patients who had one breast removed because of breast cancer, only to have the biochemical energy of cancer spread to the other breast. Jaffe noticed that if the second breast was removed, the cancer often moved to the uterus. It is not uncommon to have cancer cells metastasize in other parts of the body, so it was interesting as to why the cancer had reoccurred in the uterus. Jaffe explains that when he looked at the overall problem from an energetic perspective, he realized that the breasts represent the nourishing aspect of the womb, and since the physical parts of the body were removed, the flow of negative energy moved to the cells of the uterus, which is clearly related in function to the breasts.

Jaffe explains that if he sees heart disease developing in a person, he sees a greenish-black shadow moving throughout the area of the heart. Once he looks deeper, he may see that this energy blockage is tied to one of the valves or arteries within the heart. He has a number of processes which can remove these blocked energy states before illness in the physical heart becomes manifest.

Jaffe has not always had this ability—it is not a "gift" he was born with but rather something that took place on a fifteen mile training hike when his vision opened, due, he says, to extreme fasting. All of a sudden he could "see auras over everything." Since then he has learned how to put this unusual gift to use, detecting disease states before they manifest organically, in his medical practice. For example, while working in Hawaii, an elderly Japanese man came into his office with slight abdominal tenderness. When Jaffe looked at his patient, he saw that the man's aura was black. Quickly, he instructed his nurse to call for an ambulance, but unfortunately the man died en route to the hospital. At this point in his life, Jaffe was only able to see energy patterns, not transform them. At a later point in his life, perhaps he would have been able to help the man save himself.

The ability of some medical intuitives to deal with chronic, degenerative illness is quite remarkable. Yet many intuitives admit that their power is limited once a physical manifestation has occurred. For example, if a bone is deformed, an intuitive may be able to alleviate the pain caused by the bone, but may not be able to actually change the shape of the bone.

Letting conventional medicine
monitor your progress!

Despite his success in energy system analysis, Jaffe believes it would be unwise for patients to seek only the advice of an intuitive. He suggests that a patient first go to a physician and discover what conventional medicine has to offer.

Along the same lines, I want to strongly recommend physician Robert Gerber's classic book *Vibrational Medicine—New Choices For Healing Ourselves.* Here Dr. Gerber talks about one of the first scientists to do advanced research in the area of energetic healing, a gerontologist by the name of Bernard Grad, working at McGill University in Montreal. Grad became interested in researching the qualities of laying on of hands psychic healing. Was there really something to a vibrational approach to healing? Was there some measurable energy exchange or was this all some psychological placebo effect? And if the technique did prove to be legitimate, could a viable scientific explanation be found for it? Grad attempted to create a model in the laboratory where he could isolate the concept of patient belief and expectation and the placebo effect. To accomplish this, he chose plants and mice as his experimental "healees." His experiments also included the phenomena of accelerated wound healing via a recognized healer.

Grad decided to work with Oscar Estabany, who was known to achieve some rather miraculous healings by means of the laying on of hands.

To test Estabany's powers, Grad created an ill plant model. Now it's well known that salt is harmful to plants. When the Romans would conquer a village, for example, they would make it a point to sow the fields with a salt solution in order to inhibit plant growth thus making the town more dependent on the Roman Empire for food—a means to lastingly control a conquered people.

In his experiment Grad divided barley seedlings into two groups. Half the group was watered with a retardant salt solution not treated by a healer. The other half was treated with a salt solution held by the psychic healer Estabany for a period of fifteen minutes. Rigorous double-blind controls were utilized. Other than Grad, the experimenters did not know which plants were exposed to healing energy and which were watered with the untreated salt solutions.

The results suggested that seeds charged by the healer-treated salt solution were greater in yield and taller in size than the untreated group. Barley seeds exposed to healer energy also showed a higher chlorophyll content. It seemed apparent to Dr. Grad that some form of intelligent healing energy emanated outward from the healer's hands through the glass container into the saltwater solution.

These experiments have since been duplicated in other scientific laboratories using the individual energy fields of different psychic healers. As an aside, Estabany and Grad discussed psychic healing and its similarity to magnetic fields. Grad did an experiment in which he spun a magnetic stirring rod that charged water with a magnetic field. He found that plants treated with water that had been exposed to magnetic energy also grew faster that those that were not.

Grad conducted another study in which he surgically removed small areas of tissue from the backs of mice and then observed how these regions healed. He found that when the healer exposed his psychic healing energy to the wounds, they healed significantly faster than when the rats were held by a lab assistant or exposed to a heating element to duplicate the thermal effect of human hands.

Grad's next experiments were designed to determine if water charged with other types of subtle energy frequencies might also improve plant growth. He decided to give jars of sealed water to patients in a psychiatric institution to hold. When water held by psychotically depressed patients was used to water barley seeds, the plants demonstrated a decided retardation in their growth rate. In other words, some form of debilitating energy frequency patterns was transmitted which inhibited plant growth. This finding is obviously of great importance for health care practitioners who work with depressed patients every day. It means they should take clinical precautions to regularly restore the energetic equilibrium in their own body while they are attempting to heal the healing-inhibiting nature of depressed patients.

Using healer-assisted energy.

Dr. Justa Smith reviewed the human implications of Dr. Grad's findings. At the time, she was conducting research on enzyme activity, and it occured to her that if one could take an enzyme normally found in human beings and expose it to healer-assisted energy, it would be an excellent way to measure scientifically the healing effect such energy has on human systems generally. Dr. Smith chose trypsin, a digestive substance produced by the stomach, for her experiment, and enlisted the healer Oscar Estabany to provide the healing energy. She found that the longer Estabany held the test tubes, the faster was the rate of enzyme reaction. Estabany had no idea exactly what he was holding. He knew only that he was doing a laying-on-of-hands on a clear test tube of solution.

Smith eventually discovered that different enzymes reacted in different ways to the energy, some speeding up and others slowing down. In a third experiment there was no change at all. These results made no sense to Dr. Smith until she looked at a biochemistry chart on her office wall which showed where these enzymes normally function in a cell. To her delight, she discovered that the change exhibited by the enzymes was in each case toward the greater overall healing and metabolic balance of the cell. There appeared to be some sort of inner intelligence of this healing energy, and although Estabany didn't know precisely where his energy came from, nor what he was trying to achieve with it, the enzymes themselves consistently responded to the energy in such a way as to promote greater healing.

Following up on these results, Dr. Smith then gave Estabany test tubes of the enzyme trypsin that had been exposed to high-intensity ultraviolet light, causing the proteins in the molecule to denature and lose their active site, so that they are no longer able to function as enzymes. She discovered that when Mr. Estabany held the test tubes, the enzymes became restructured and re-patterned, regained their active state, and began to function normally. As in Grad's experiments, the longer he held them, the faster the enzymes worked. This ability to cause a system to move to states of increased order and organization is quite remarkable, as is the idea that the enzymes were accelerated in a fashion similar to the effect of the high-intensity magnetic fields. An important fact is that the new level of healing activity sustained itself over time.

During this period, researchers tried to measure the actual magnetic fields emitted from the hands of healers which seemed to be magnetic in substance. However, with the equipment available at the time, they were unable to detect energy fields that would be of the intensity required to get these same effects shown in healer-accelerated enzymes. Empirical evidence suggested that a gifted healer's touch was no longer an abstraction but an instrument of healing that was similar in nature to magnetic fields but could not be measured by conventional electromagnetic field recording devices. Also evident was that some healers had the ability to actually facilitate a restructuring and overall healing and organizational effect on enzyme systems and that this healer-exposed life energy seemed to have its own innate natural healing wisdom.

Bioenergetic research

Justa Smith, another scientist working with energetic healers, began to wonder what actually took place when these healers did a laying-on-of-hands on water. How was this water altered so that it was able to somehow biologically accelerate plant growth? She found that in healer-augmented water, a significant change in the hydrogen bonding of the water molecules took place. Water is made up of two hydrogen and one oxygen atom. It is a polar molecule in that it has a slightly positive and a slightly negative end. The positive ends of one water molecule tend to line up with the negative ends of other water molecules. This structure is referred to as surface tension. Experimental evidence suggests that the energetic field circling the healer's hands alters the water's molecular bonding and changes the surface tension of water.

Is distant healing possible?

Dr. Robert Miller, a research chemist, worked extensively with two famous spiritual healers, Olga Worrell and her husband,

Ambrose Worrell. They not only could bioenergetically heal by a laying-on-of-hands, or by placing their hands at a slight distance from a patient's body, but they could accomplish the same results by simply focusing prayer thoughts on a particular patient, often at a great distance.

Olga Worell could influence the growth rate of targeted seedlings from a remote place in the laboratory. More astounding still was the fact that when Olga and Ambrose sent vibrational healing frequencies to the laboratory from their home in Baltimore, some six hundred miles away, at the exact moment they were holding the rye grass in their thoughts, its growth rate jumped by more than 800 percent. When they stopped energizing the plants, the growth rate dropped to only 200 percent above normal—though it never returned to normal. It seems that such healing energies have negative entropic properties (growth-promoting capacity) and are independent of distance—and that all life is one and connected. In this way such energies differ from conventional electromagnetic fields, which decrease as they dimensionally move away from their source. This school of thought strongly suggests that what is being dealt with here are higher multidimensional energy frequencies that move beyond the speed of light.

Inducing healing energies via therapeutic touch.

D r. Delores Krieger, professor of nursing at New York University, after reviewing the aforementioned experiments on plant life, mouse wounds, and enzymatic activity, became determined to learn whether she could get the same measure of healing effects in human beings. Krieger once again enlisted the aid of Oscar Estabany, asking him to come out to a farm outside of New York. They collected two groups of patients with a variety of different illnesses. Krieger established a control group that spent time out in the sunlight, while the other half spent a little time each day with Estabany receiving laying-on-of-hands healing treatment.

Now, hemoglobin in human beings is biochemically similar to the chlorophyll molecule, with the exception that it has an iron atom present at its center rather than magnesium. Krieger theorized that if healers could increase plant chlorophyll, they might also be able to increase a patient's blood hemoglobin level. Following the experiment researchers analyzed the two groups of patients, one healer-treated and the other untreated, and found that the healer's treatments had improved the health of the patients who had recieved it, and specifically raised their blood hemoglobin levels.

This was wonderful news, and it helped to explain why cancer patients who have undergone a laying on of hands healing treatment have occasionally demonstrated elevated hemoglobin levels in spite of exposure to agents that suppress bone marrow which, as a rule, induce lower hemoglobin levels.

An excellent book on the subject is *Massage: The Ultimate Illustrated Guide* by Clare Maxwell-Hudson. It covers Swedish, Chinese, Indian, Shiatsu and Moroccan massage.

Another alternative healing modality was discovered during Dr. Krieger's study. It was found that Estabany was able to charge not only water with healing energy which could help reverse illness, but also cotton and wool dressings. It was found that patients could actually feel bioenergetic vibrations emanating from the dressings (which contained stored healer-assisted energy) as they were placed next to their bodies. The result: a vast improvement in patient physiologic states and symptom disappearance in a large percentage of healer-treated patients.

The next question Krieger asked was whether there was a

way to teach *others* how to induce healing energies (a kind of therapeutic partnership) to create physiologic change in patients? Can someone acquire this skill or are people born with it? To answer this question, she conducted experiments with clairvoyant and healer Dora van Gelder Kunz (who worked with physician Karagulla). Together they created a course to teach healing to nursing students. They called it "Therapeutic Touch" and it initially was taught by Kunz. They found that hands-on healing was bioenergetically helpful in a wide assortment of cases. Incidentally, their experiments included healing animals as well.

Therapeutic touch can be learned!

The real test came when Kunz and Krieger trained health care professionals in a multi-hospital study which compared the effects of therapeutic touch on patients' hemoglobin levels. The study showed that people who were instructed in therapeutic touch were also able to elevate hemoglobin levels in patients. What this tells us is that therapeutic touch and bioenergetic healing are not necessarily innate human skills. They can be learned, and we all have a great inner potential for healing.

In simple terms, you might think of therapeutic touch as being somewhat similar to the effect of a jumper cable. Think of energy transfer via a jumper cable channeled from a strong battery to a weaker battery, somewhat like recharging a person's battery. Another way of looking at the phenomenon is that healers are transmitting an etheric life force energy, a negative entropic magnetic energy that has inherent healing wisdom which seems to know where in the physical body to go in the meridian systems to energetically rebalance the Chakras.

Believing is seeing!

I was first introduced in 1995 to Dr. Robert Jaffe's advanced healing techniques when a friend sent me an audiotape describing his medical practice. The tape (free by calling 1-888-USA-SUFI) contained an interview with Jaffe by well-known psychologist Larry Jensen who related the remarkable experiences of his own daughter, his mother, and three medical doctors, all of whom had been successfully treated by Jaffe. After listening to the tape, I remained somewhat skeptical, finding it difficult to accept that such anecdotal "evidence" was entirely true. The rigorous experiments by Grad, Smith, and Miller brought me around, and I came to accept that such healing was within the realm of possibility. The paranormal events I myself had experienced also helped me to open my mental receptor sites to such possibilities.

After listening to Jaffe's tape and then reading his interview with author Paul Farini in a past issue of *Miracles Magazine* (now out-of-print), I decided to call Jaffe directly and try to get a healing over the telephone. That's right; he can actually heal over the telephone. Or so his secretary claimed. I had read that C. Norman Shealy, M.D., Ph.D., a neurosurgeon formerly at Harvard working with Carolyn Myss, had stated that studies showed she was 93 percent accurate in her diagnoses of patients over the telephone, up to twelve hundred miles away, given only the patients' names. It seems that Jaffe, too, can intuitively perceive the presence and nature of a disease state within a person's physical body—at a distance—by "seeing" their mental, emotional and spiritual life force or energetic life history.

My own reasons for calling Jaffe were twofold. In the first place, I myself had been diagnosed with a malignant tumor, and I did want a healing. But I also wanted to interview the doctor because I was considering writing a book about medical intuitives. All I can say about my telephone "reading" with Jaffe was he was the first person who got right down into the very core of my soul. I call it "soul-to-soul" work. On the strength of this conversation, I decided to attend one of his workshops and see with my own eyes just how he uses a powerful new form of healing that includes the best of allopathic, energetic, and spiritually-based healing.

The workshop I attended in Minneapolis included twenty-six people—twenty-six potential "miracles," you might say. I had no idea what to expect, but I had a compelling desire to meet Jaffe. It was like an inner summons. After all, if he could help me move mountains over the telephone, maybe his curriculum, a blending of the conventional and the unconventional, could guide me down a more transformative, spiritually-energetic healing path.

There is little question that I was searching for a second chance at life, which I hoped to gain from Jaffe's workshop. But I was becoming more and more aware that I would have to open myself willfully to the potential for healing in every aspect of my life, mental, spiritual, intellectual, emotional, and physical. I was ready to make that commitment, because I was beginning to believe that cancer was a wake-up call telling me that my soul was seeking a healing peace that would change me and also the world around me—a peace that had been lacking prior to my cancer diagnosis.

Many of Jaffe's workshop attendees were therapists from around the country who came to learn Jaffe's new healing process so they could incorporate it into their own medical practices. And there is no question that after spending almost fifty hours with Jaffe and my fellow attendees, I deemed them sensible and responsible professionals to the Nth degree. Like me, some were skeptical and hard-nosed, having come from a purely scientific, rather conventional background. Other health care providers were there also, as well as teachers, nuns, and just plain spiritual seekers. Talk about diversity! All races, colors, and religions were represented. Perhaps the one thing we all had in common was an inquiring mind. And as Jaffe led us on our individual journeys, you could feel the vibratory transmission of love consciousness throughout all aspects of the workshop.

The first day of the workshop.

This session opened with Jaffe telling us his story. He explained how he left the field of traditional medicine after a successful eight-year practice, to study acupuncture, homeopathy, and electro-acupuncture, and he described the afternoon when, following a fifteen-mile hike, he had first seen auras, which subsequently prompted his investigation of energy auras and their relationship with illness. He described how, on one occasion, he had impulsively released his pent-up rage at the established medical system by actually screaming, and unintentionally ridding his body of a debilitating eye infection that had left him blind:

When I released the anger and was willing to see it, that's when the eye healed. Then I knew that this was the way I wanted to practice medicine. I wanted to use auric vision to teach people what was causing their disease.

For the next five years, I worked with thousands of people. I'd put them in front of a white board and I would look at their auras. I'd see where in the field it was black, where it was light, where it was dark red, and so on. Then I'd do a deep history of their disease, and try to determine what was going on in their lives when they got sick. Putting all this information together, I actually developed a system that was workable and teachable. And that became Advanced Energy Healing. The system worked. We were getting 80 to 90 percent success from virtually everybody who walked in the door, including people with cancer and MS.

Learning heart-centered healing

That first day Jaffe gave an overview of the basic concepts behind his own healing strategies, how he healed, and how we could, too. It was a blending of the purely scientific and the mystical, like vicariously attending medical school at an ashram. The concepts were really quite simple and made perfect sense. In fact, they resonated on every level of my consciousness. They would, I could sense, take time to assimilate, however. Jaffe emphasized the heart Chakra energies through which all love flows and explained how all of us can channel those energies to transform our past wounds and promote the healing process.

The essence of Jaffe's workshop:

Time after time, Jaffe intuitively put at our fingertips the information essential for identifying an underlying emotional disorder and determining the best approaches for diagnosis, treatment, and follow up. His Advanced Energy Healing program is a clear systematic healing process that walks you through what you need to know to begin to heal at every plane of your being.

Jaffe repeatedly pointed out four essential factors to healing and living a more creative and productive life:

1. God gives us experiences to provide us spiritual growth.
2. There is always a spiritual lesson present in crisis that we need to learn.
3. To heal, we must be in the deep presence of God Consciousness.
4. By anchoring in God (love), deep change can occur.

When a patient is unwilling to connect with God, Consciousness, Jaffe states, he finds it difficult to heal that person.

"I can help you heal," he says, "but you must be truthful to your-self, acknowledge what is taking place in your life, walk forward, and close the door behind you." The highest healing takes place, he says, when an individual courageously embraces self-aware-ness, self-assessment, self-understanding, and love. Embracing self-awareness without actually connecting with God-conscious-ness (love) just won't do it, Jaffe says.

Emotional, psychological and spiritual breakthrough via a problem-based approach.

On the second day of the workshop, Jaffe asked for volun-teers to work with him in furthering their own healing pro-cesses. Invariably, he chose for transformation those volunteers with the most difficult disease states. This was obvious because of the nature of the questions these people had asked the day before. In the course of time, I witnessed individuals begin to be healed from a wide spectrum of diseases for which conventional medicine had failed to find a solution. What was notable was that never once did Jaffe back away from a complex challenge. With compassion, humanity, and an exuberant spirit, he met each individual circumstance head-on, all the while demystifying the dynamics of precisely how he heals and how virtually all of us can achieve similar transformative results. It was an inspiring medical Grand Rounds lesson that is seldom witnessed outside a hospital environment. That he was correct in his perceptive appraisals and insightful solutions was proven in one case after another.

Because of Jaffe's expert medical and intuitive guidance in highlighting concise and usable energy healing points during the workshop proceedings, I found myself able to shift my perspective and reevaluate my life priorities (emotional and spiritual "issues") and apply his healing methods to them. His numerous case studies—real-world vignettes—focused on and demonstrated his key healing principles in action.

Volunteers willing to take charge of their lives.

It should be pointed out that Jaffe healed volunteers who were willing to take charge of their lives and assist him as a partner in the healing process. These were individuals who understood that the key impetus in change is being able to respond to crisis by challenging life's obstacles that interfere with mental and spiritual growth. Noting this, Jaffe helped each volunteer look inward, identify and reframe his or her toxic energy field (excessive fears, unfinished business, and other obstructions preventing spiritual development), release it, and then enlist God's healing energy.

Jaffe teaches that God is not a particular religion, nor is He an intermediary. God is God. And He should be contacted directly through prayer. According to Jaffe, to heal mentally, emotionally, spiritually and physically, what is required is deep introspection and the self-determination to heal yourself, since change can emerge only if you dissolve yourself into God-consciousness (love). To choose to remain stuck in the toxic energy of anger, resentment, et al., for example, only delays healing, Jaffe says. Closure of past wounds and unfinished emotional business is therefore essential to the healing process since they can continue to cause physical dysfunction.

Some real life examples of how Jaffe can raise the probability of healing in emotional, spiritual, and physical terms

Example #1: Suppressed Anger

There were several nuns in our workshop. When Jaffe asked for a volunteer to help illustrate his healing process, one nun stated that she had an unresolved emotional issue that had reigned within her consciousness for more than fifty years. Her sister (to whom she had been extremely close) had died at the age of six. Jaffe's insight: "And from then on, you've been unable to forgive God. And that's the deeply-entrenched emotional issue you must resolve."

Even though it was scary for the nun to honor her issue and go to the place where the open wound was living (even with Jaffe's intuitive skills), she was willing to choose self-responsibility and change. With Jaffe's help, she was able to explain the root cause of her consuming negative energy and release it, so that her trust in God could return. What I found equally interesting was the nun's absolute trust in Jaffe to enter and heal her victim space. Using his "release-of-toxic-energy" healing formula (explained below), patiently, with compassion and love, he didn't let her down.

At the end of the session, in order to further unblock the negative emotions that had been controlling her for so many years, we all invoked a healing prayer for the nun, from the Creator. It was a moving and inspiring event, showing how a circle of love can be immensely empowering and therapeutic. Watching the nun move from a position of low ebb to revitalization was mind-altering. I began to realize that (a) in our daily life choices we create our own negative perceptions and consequences; (b) if we live in love, we attract love to us (the opposite is true as well); (c) the energy of love can heal virtually any victim energy pattern. The entire episode was like watching the energy release of hot lava from an erupting volcano. You could feel the love in the room releasing and replacing the toxic energy that had been lurking as rage in the nun's inner being for so many years. It was apparent to all of us that living in love (opening your heart to all people—with no distinction), can quite literally reorganize a toxic energy field, leaving the soul to resonate with the deep love of God. Perhaps, I thought, enlightenment or illuminated knowing is nothing more than looking at life with the eye of the heart (the spirituality of deep love). The life lesson: Like attracts like. Anger and self-pity contaminate your energy field and stifle the healing process. The truth remains: Deep love heals.

Example #2: Chronic Fatigue

In another workshop, a volunteer exhibited a dense red field that was giving him chronic fatigue syndrome. With compassion and love, Jaffe showed the man how to release the shutdown emotional energy that was underlying his disease and affecting his immune system. Jaffe closed his eyes, scanned the man's energy field, activated it to move, asked him several defining questions about the color and sound of the energy field, and then showed the attendee how to create healing by releasing the pent-up noxious energy he was harboring within. (See Jaffe's "release-of-toxic-energy" formula below.)

After about twenty minutes, the man's pulsating chronic fatigue energy disappeared and his complexion changed from pasty white to a cherubic youthfulness. Under Jaffe's guidance, the volunteer had released his stressful negative energy by directly facing and reevaluating a past emotional trauma (deep resentment at being abandoned by his parents). He admitted that for the first time in many, many years, he didn't feel tired and depressed. Jaffe had established an environment within which the patient could move forward in his life and no longer deny what he knew to be true—that toxic emotions had been contaminating and controlling it. This change in direction and outlook had an immediate impact on his health and well-being.

Example #3: Fourth-Stage Uterine Cancer

A more complex case that Jaffe recounted concerned a woman whose uterine cancer had spread throughout her abdomen and into the colon. Her doctors had given her about six weeks to live and she was close to dying. Jaffe "saw" that her abdomen was filled with red, toxic energy, and uncovered the fact that her father had sexually abused her. Worse than that, her testimony had been instrumental in convicting him, and he was soon to be released from a fifteen-year jail term. The woman was terrified. When this toxic energy was released, she stopped bleeding—the first time in six months—and the cancer was gone.

It reappeared three months later, however. The woman had taken a job as a waitress in a bar, and she often seduced men into giving her larger tips. This misuse of her sexuality had reanimated the toxic energy. Jaffe once again helped her release her controlling emotions and recharge her energy fields, the cancer again left—but not for long. She started having multiple sexual relationships. Jaffe explored even more deeply and found that, in previous lives, the woman had been a geisha girl and a male pedophile (if you don't believe in the principle of afterlife, there is no question that this story will push your ability to believe). By the way, the first to bring the concept of reincarnation to my attention was Edgar Cayce, the famous medical intuitive. As William A. McGarey, M.D. so aptly described the doctrine, Cayce "saw" each of us as an eternal being, having existed in a form that is self-conscious prior to birth and continuing that existence when the physical body dies. The life lesson: In this lifetime, according to Jaffe, her father had reflected what she had been. When she faced this issue directly, her immune system responded and her cancer disappeared.

"If love is the answer" says Jaffe, "what's the question?"

Over and over, Jaffe stressed that God Consciousness is love and love is resolution. It's giving without expectation. It's understanding that love connects and that love-energy nurtures. It's selfless. It's forgiveness. Offer it freely, and it'll return many fold. Love strengthens, inspires, and bonds. Love lightens your burdens. It changes others. Even in intolerable situations, God's love can free you, says Jaffe. Such are the healing wonders of deep love.

Jaffe's "release-of-toxic-energy" healing formula.

In its most simplistic form, Jaffe's healing "formula" goes something like this:

1. *First, determine the emotions behind your particular illness.* For example, if you have a life-threatening illness and Jaffe helps you clear out your toxic energy field, this is only a temporary condition, unless you clear up the ongoing emotional issue that has caused the disease in the first place. In my own case, Jaffe said I needed to work on spiritual blocks, which he felt I was now in the process of unlocking and resolving. I knew he was on target, for I had formerly been an agnostic (a very large lifetime investment

on my part), and the workshop was the beginning of my walk to becoming a deist. It's a path I needed to move on to heal mind, body, and spirit. By looking into my energy field, Jaffe told me he could see this energy hindrance in the right side of my face—the exact area cancer had been detected. He also stated the cancer was my wake-up call to move on a more spiritual and loving path. In order to remove the spiritual disturbance in the energy field, he said, I needed to understand and clear up the destructive energy or core spiritual issue that initially had created my disease.

2. *Visualize the disease as energy patterns (obstacles) whose hold you want to release.* According to Jaffe, there's always a psycho-emotional component that creates a pattern of energy that changes the physical body and underlies disease. It's this specific, subtle energy pattern moving through you that Jaffe can see and help you clear, thus enabling you to heal. Acupuncture, cranial-sacral work, and spiritual messaging can help alter negative energy fields, but he reiterated over and over that if you don't clear the underlying psycho-emotional or psycho-spiritual issue behind the disease, it can recur.

Once you take charge of your medical journey by reclaiming your inner and outer health, you'll never see the universe the same again. You'll find, as others have, that there is a power higher than a physician that still makes house calls.

Chapter 8

How to Plan Coincidence
to Suit Yourself

While on vacation, my wife Joanie, some friends and I, decided to seek out our favorite diversion, a flea market. Knowing that I enjoy wandering around by myself, we agreed to meet at a specific booth at a precise time. Being that it was one of the largest flea markets in the world, somehow I got lost and was late in arriving at the designated spot. When I got there, the others were nowhere in sight. Intuitively, I felt a strong guiding impulse telling me to go to a specific booth owned by friends that was located a good distance away. Trusting my nature, even though it did not follow the dictates of logic (which would have meant remaining where I was until the others appeared), I quickly left our meeting place and proceeded to the distant booth. There, awaiting my presence were Joanie and the others. It turns out that she had just remarked quite seriously to her friends, "I have no idea where Sid is, so hold on a minute while I shut my eyes and send him a clear message telling him we're at this booth." To everyone's total amazement, the message was mystically communicated to my inner senses. Trusting and following my inner impulses, I had taken immediate action and consequently, I achieved the desired outcome.

Seeking congruity between your mind and heart

Events like these happen to me often because I've learned to trust and rely heavily on my subjective reality—my inner impulses. Though such "hunches" may seem illogical, by heeding them, and listening to your inner consciousness, you will transcend conventional mental barriers and open up new avenues upon which to move forward on your healing path. What I've found true over many years of experience is that by acting upon, rather than ignoring, my deepest impulses I have rarely made a poor life decision. But this is assuming that congruity clearly exists between my mind and heart. When my mind says one thing and my heart another, I become wary and sense very quickly that I am "off path." When they're in total agreement, however, I sense intuitively that I am "on path."

Having an open-ended system of beliefs

In the flea market example, I could easily have ignored my intuition regarding wife's whereabouts and done the "sensible" thing by staying put. I believe that the postive outcome was the result of my open-ended belief system which accepts telepathy as a natural form of communication. This open-endedness expands my sphere of creativity, making it easier to respond to stimuli that arrive in unusual ways. Allowing my receptor sites to remain open—rather than questioning their validity—all the while confidently expecting the outcome I strongly desire to take place, tends to expand my psychic consciousness wide enough to perceive higher forms of being.

In *The Individual and the Nature of Mass Events*, by Jane Roberts, the chief character, Seth, says that inner "impulses are the language of the psyche." Nevertheless, most people are constricted by beliefs that view communication of thought impulses, as virtually impossible.

Elevating your total bodily health.

Many people construct mental frameworks (beliefs) that largely shut out the possibility of intuitive impulses. With that single choice, they effectively reduce the quality of their life. When you allow belief-impediments to obstruct your path, and even perceive them to be immovable, rather than making an effort to clear them away, it validates your prejudiced belief that "life is only one obstacle after another." Did you recognize the voice of victimhood in that statement? Individuals holding firm to that feeling tend to get exactly what they focus on, because they have arbitrarily closed off all avenues to development and end up feeling powerless and downtrodden. There are few internal messages that can crack through a wall of this kind of negativity. Yet people who cling to such non-assertive beliefs and feelings end up shutting down their internal machinery. The toxic chemical reaction they set in motion in their body is a result of their deep-seated beliefs, thoughts and feelings.

Inner world under repair.

When you're faced with a serious life challenge, it's important that you mobilize all of the inner tools you can muster. Certainly, the impulses of despair and powerlessness are not among the resources you should dial into, since victimhood unchecked can only reduce that quality of your life. The information available to intuition far surpasses knowledge gained through the intellect—which takes most of its information from external reality. My belief is that we all have access—call it genetic programming if you will—to experience understanding on an intuitive level. The first step to re-familiarizing yourself with this powerful source of information and inspiration will be to allow such experiences into your framework of beliefs. Using intuitive impulses wisely, and trusting them, will allow you to get in touch with Infinite Energy—an ever-expanding power always at your disposal that can sustain mind, body, and spirit.

Contradictory impulses.

As stated earlier, when I make life decisions, I'm aware of the internal dialogue between my heart and mind. In confronting a problem, if my mind tells me to take a particular path and my heart is not in complete agreement, I know I'm off the "path" I was meant to take. For example, one day I was asked by a local physician to get involved full time in a nutritional supplement project. In reviewing the situation, I concluded it was indeed a most worthwhile project. My mind advised me to get immersed in the project but my heart warned that such involvement would detract from my true mission in life, which I believe is conducting workshops for those with chronic illnesses. Since congruity between my mind and my heart was conspicuously absent, I decided to devote minimum time to the project. It was astonishing the amount of energy I had tied up in making the decision, which, as you already know, can be detrimental to the entire back-to-wellness process. When I finally did make a decision, however, I could actually feel the blocked energy (stress)—a chemical reaction—release from my body.

I now make virtually all my life decisions by seeking congruity (harmony) between mind and heart. At the same time, I've become sensitive to an inner dialogue through which I process and resolve contradictory impulses. To a high degree, this requires trusting the deep spontaneous messages that surface from your subconscious and noting where unity exists. The operative word is *trusting*. It is my belief that these internal messages emanate from Infinite Power and are vital to one's well-being. I view them as valid messages meant to provide directions (much like a map) that I should follow, in order to stay on a healing path of self-realization.

Give your intuitive messages a fair hearing.

But you can't receive life-enhancing messages if your receptor sites are closed or if you choose to deny them validity. By disallowing the expression of your inner impulses, you curb future growth in all areas of your life.

Chapter Nine

How to Change Negative Feelings in Seconds!

First things first:

All negative feelings (vibrational energy in motion) start with YOU focusing your thoughts and feelings on DON'T WANTS!

Let's see if you recognize some (ugh!) everyday examples:

I don't want to be sick.
I don't want to be in a bad relationship.
I don't want to be unable to pay my bills on time.
I don't want to work for my miserable boss.
I don't want to deal with tough customers.
I don't want to come down with the flu.
I don't want to go to work today.
I don't want to be held up at gunpoint.
I don't want to feel guilty.

One thing for sure: Think in terms of DON'T WANTS and you're definitely not going to feel good about your focus—and that's guaranteed!

Want some more examples that you won't feel good about? Here then are more negative (bad-feeling) vibrations that, unless discarded, you can be certain will bring back matching life experiences into some aspect of your life:

If only I had been brought up rich.

If only I had a better job.

If only my parents had treated me better.

If only I had better friends and relatives.

If only people would stop talking behind my back.

If only I could afford better clothes.

If only I could afford a new computer.

If only I could stop drinking.

If only I could stop arguing with people.

If only other people would stop driving so dangerously.

If only my kids would stop using alcohol and drugs.

If only my kids would get better grades.

If only people would give me more respect.

If only I were more popular.

If only I could do my own thing.

If only I could stand up for what I really believe.

If only I cared less about what my friends think.

If only I would start doing things I like and not what others want for me.

If only I had stayed in school.

If only I hadn't married so early.

If only I could get to my appointment on time.

If only I had a better marriage.

If only my family would approve what I want to do.

Etcetera. Etcetera. Etcetera. Talk about locking yourself into a framework of negative thoughts and feelings!

Here are even more thinly disguised negative (bad-feeling) vibrations people choose to focus on and empower, which bring more of the same future negative events into their lives? (Remember: Like attracts like.)

I really want to get back to wellness.

I really want to be able to pay my bills on time.

I really want to lose some weight.

I really want to stop smoking now.

I really want to feel safe in this city.

I really want my marriage to get a whole lot better.

I really want to get a better job.

I really want my spouse, significant other or
    partner to make more money.

I really want to get promoted.

Would you agree "really want" thoughts and feelings are a potent remedy to humankind's ills? Not! Here's why: "Where's the focus?" Where's the sensation of exuberant emotion? Where's the vibrancy of spirit? Where's pulsating energy flowing? Where's expansiveness? Where's conscious intent? Where's confidence? Where's momentum?

Pretty obvious, isn't it?

The focus is on insufficiency, on inadequacy, on DON'T WANTS! The result: You experience what you focus on!

The thing is, how can "really want" people ever achieve what they *really* want when what they're thinking makes them FEEL bad? The more you find yourself focusing on "really wants" with strong emotion, the more you give vibrating thought-energy the right to enter your life as matching events in time and space.

The corrective action: Since what you vibrate on you get, STOP sending out invitations of what you DON'T WANT. By focusing on sending out magnetic energy of what you DO WANT, you'll begin matching up with WANT vibrations on the same frequency.

Can you now see why it's so important to identify and monitor your Don't Wants? It's to learn to focus intention and positive thought-and-feeling-energy on the experiences you DO WANT to bring into your life.

One of my all-time favorite books, is *Excuse Me, Your Life is Waiting* by Lynn Grabhorn. In a sense, she has been a channeled-in companion in writing parts of this chapter. I suggest you read her book—several times if necessary!

Okay, here is where we have a little heart-to-heart about

HOW TO DELETE AND REPLACE DON'T WANTS:

1. See yourself as a joyful conscious creator with good reason for being.
2. Quickly replace your DON'T WANTS with WANTS.
3. Each day, mentally challenge the limits of your physical reality.

Since thoughts and feelings create like events, below are some *before* and *after* examples of how to intentionally, excitingly, and effortlessly tune into the vibrations of good-feeling thoughts which, as a result, will create more of the same.

Please note the Before examples represent pre-conceived, habitually-used and defective assumptions that cut you off from Source Energy, and thus are likely to generate feelings of powerlessness. By contrast, After examples get you vibrating in a highly empowering manner that draws to you the desired event(s) you want to experience. Are you ready? Okay, let's get started setting your mind at ease:

Before: I don't want to be sick.
 After: Every day in every way I'll THINK and FEEL perfectly healthy.

Before: I don't want to be in a bad relationship.
 After: Every day in every way I'll THINK what a good relationship FEELS like.

Before: I don't want to be unable to pay my bills.
 After: Every day in every way I'll THINK and FEEL what it's like to KNOW I can pay all my bills.

Before: I don't want to work for a miserable boss.
 After: Every day in every way I'll THINK and FEEL exactly what's it's like to work for a great boss.

Before: I don't want to deal with difficult people.
 After: Every day in every way I'll THINK and FEEL what it's like to win over so-called difficult people.

Before: I don't want to come down with the flu.
 After: Every day in every way I'll THINK and FEEL healthy, regardless of what others around me perceive.

Before: I don't want to go to work today.

   After: Every day in every way I'll THINK and FEEL great KNOWING that I consciously create my day.

Before: I don't seem to laugh as much as I used to.

   After: Every day in every way I'll THINK and FEEL the joyous nature of my spontaneous self.

Before: I don't want to be held up at gun point.

   After: Every day in every way I'll THINK and FEEL totally safe.

Before: I don't want to feel guilty.

   After: Every day in every way I'll THINK and FEEL free of morally judging others.

Note #1:

As you switch your mental focus from Before to After thoughts, FEEL vibrations of excitement. FEEL vibrations of enthusiasm. This double action tends to reinforce and hasten the formation of the events you want to enter your life.

Note #2:

Be aware that your present negative circumstances are the consequences of a past focus on harmful and self-limiting thoughts and feelings that you can only change in the present.

Note #3:

If you find yourself resisting feeling-good thought-vibrations, by all means ask yourself, "What central thoughts, beliefs, and expectations are behind my resistance?"

Right about now you may be thinking, "I still don't believe this stuff really works." If so, then perhaps it would be worthwhile reminding yourself *why* you're seeking to escape your bubble of negative belief. Take a good hard look at the potential fallout if you persist in choosing thoughts and feelings that inhibit and restrict you from consciously creating what you want in life. How will you ever know unparalleled achievements unless you give new, healthier thoughts and feelings your best effort (by the way, the word "try" is not in my vocabulary!)

More to the point: Do you ever notice people who seem to get stuck focusing on misery? They play depressing music, mope around not doing much of anything and exhibit body language that radiates anything but well-being—you know the scene. Notice as well how their voice projects a sense of joylessness, which mirrors their thoughts and feelings? The whole scene is almost too morbid to contemplate.

This brings me to this single question quiz, "for your eyes only." I promise it will stimulate your imagination and launch you on the path of self-empowerment right this very moment. Ready? Here's the single question: *What would you say are the most important ingredients behind deliberately forming your life experiences?* No, it's not "a jug of wine, a loaf of bread and thou beside me singing in the wilderness." The answer is:

THINKING, FEELING and KNOWING that JOY is your natural birthright; your absolute right!

This capstone message on seeking joyfulness and coloring outside the lines reminds me of an inspiring saying I once saw inscribed on a T-Shirt. It says, "Maybe God has bigger plans for you than you have for yourself."

When you change your focus and start flowing energy in new and healthier ways, it allows you to magnetically attract what you vibrate. On the other hand, by continuing to follow those familiar but unhealthy currents of negative thought and feeling, you shut off your connection to Source Energy.

So, if toxic thoughts and feelings are getting in the way of your life, the rather obvious question is, Why not use your innate ability as a deliberate creator to create what you want, without having to justify your effervescent feelings to someone else? If you focus on what you want while all the while resonating with the vibrations of the golden rule, you definitely are on purpose, which, in my opinion, is where each of us ought to be as spiritual beings.

Chapter Ten

Is It Now Possible to Create Your Own Internal Anti-depressant Chemicals That Make You Feel Good?

Has a new daily strategy to restore calmness and well-being been found at last?

What is there about some people that makes them so much happier than others? Is it possible that somehow they are creating their own feeling-good chemicals? Before we get to that, I'd like to ask you another question. What is the one thing in all of nature that often brings about its own suffering? Assuming the new science, quantum physics is correct in suggesting that there is no reality until it is perceived reality, the answer is:

Inertia!

Since your feelings mirror your thoughts, when you wallow in a state of helplessness and hopelessness, and perceive yourself as a victim of your life circumstances, you're likely to attract more of the same. The solution? Cast inertia aside, and let go of old fear-based notions, so that you can begin to manufacture your own anti-depressant chemicals, thus positively affecting virtually every cell and vital organ in your body.

By cultivating positive mental imagery, and directing your energy toward beneficial thoughts and feelings (think, molecules of emotion), you can raise and direct vibrational energy to improve the climate of your inner reality. In so doing, you'll find that you can alter your mood, reduce anxiety and stress, and boosts immune system functioning. You have this ability. I have it. Everyone has it.

Want a case in point? Well, laughter is a good example of an instant high that can induce feelings of well-being. Zen Buddhists believe that laughing for merely ten minutes is equal in therapeutic effect to six hours of deep meditation. In his book, *Anatomy of an Illness*, Norman Cousins cited instance after instance of the power of laughter to cure what the scientific community had diagnosed as an incurable illness. He discovered that just fifteen minutes of laughter allowed him to be pain and drug-free for several hours. The explanation: It appears laughter elevates the body's natural painkillers. Another example showing the effects of the release of good-feeling chemicals is the movie *Patch Adams*, which also displayed the powerful affects of laughter therapy.

The physician William Fry, formerly of Stanford University, has observed that laughter can offer a significant body workout that not only makes you feel good, thus reducing stress, but elevates oxygen levels in the blood. Perhaps you have noticed yourself that laughter gives a sudden vitalizing boost that can change an energy-depleting mindset into inner peace. At a cellular level, it's not unlike taking an anti-depressant drug without the attending cost or side effects.

In light of these facts, it would definitely be worthwhile whenever possible, to limit your use of conventional medications, and begin to explore the unlimited forces of your own psyche.

Your challenge: To teach your brain to make its own anti-depressant drugs.

Science is now telling us that a good belly laugh elevates the level of immunoglobulin A, which boosts the body's basic defenses on a molecular level. Simply put, daily doses of laughter are a very powerful healing force that can actually activate the wellness process.

Having fun can bring about changes in your body chemistry.

Let's say you just love taking roller coaster rides at amusement parks. It's your passion. You simply can't get enough of it. You see it as just plain old-fashioned fun. (By the way, your fun passion could also be walking, singing, skiing, golf, tennis, sewing, gardening, or whatever.) You may not be aware that at the moment when you're having loads of fun, your body is manufacturing Interferon and Interleukin—chemicals that are highly potent anti-cancer drugs. On the other hand, if you're a wannabe race car driver but are highly fearful of the sport, your body will manufacture the chemicals adrenalin and cortisol, both of which can be harmful to immune system functioning. In short, your body is an apothecary more powerful by far than any drug store on the planet.

Ever wonder what's happening internally when you're unruffled and calm practicing yoga or meditation? Would you believe your body is busy manufacturing molecules similar to those found in the drug valium?

Can you actually go about making good-feeling chemicals?

The answer is Yes! You can consciously and deliberately raise the serotonin and norepinephrine levels in your brain. These two chemicals are neurotransmitters—chemical substances released from nerve fibers that affect the transfer of an impulse to another nerve or muscle. A shortage or excess of either one may lead to stress, anxiety, depression, ADHD, and bipolar disorder.

Norepinephrine is a neurotransmitter similar to adrenaline. High levels of norepinephrine can cause unfriendly behavior. For example, if, at an early age, you had to deal with excessive amounts of stress, you could have acquired a permanent deficiency in serotonin and high levels of norepinephrine, which can lead to bouts of hostile behavior in later life.

The nervous system responds to acute stress by releasing norepinephrine and epinephrine (adrenaline), which elevate the heart rate and blood pressure by launching an individual into their natural fight or flight defense mode.

In depression, levels of neurotransmitters such as serotonin are usually low. The class of drugs called Selective Serotonin Reuptake Inhibitors (SSRIs) are used to treat depression, anxiety disorders, and some personality disorders, by allowing the body to make the *best* use of the reduced amounts of serotonin it has at any given instant. In time, the levels of natural serotonin will once again elevate and, in some instances, a SSRI drug can be reduced and withdrawn.

Once again, we return to the question:

Can you write a different daily life script by actually manipulating your brain cells so you feel better?

Yes, by focusing on new, healthy thoughts and feelings, you can raise your serotonin and norepinephrine levels, which will make you feel better. This elevation in mood, in turn, will lead to more positive experiences in your daily life, thus reaffirming the positive imaging that lies at the root of it all.

Your assignment is to use the following simple strategy to manage your brain cells (incidentally, always allow your physician to monitor your progress): While maintaining an inner and outer smile, either before, during, or after you are mentally visualizing whatever outcome you want to achieve, visualize both serotonin and norepinephrine (happy molecules) gushing through your bloodstream to all the cells in your body.

As you practice this exercise, you'll be creating your own high-frequency, good-feeling chemicals. In a sense, this is what antidepressant drugs achieve by raising the level of serotonin and norepinephrine in your brain. The brain's natural endorphins act to alleviate pain, causing feelings of pleasure and sleepiness. Extensive aerobic exercise is also known to release endorphins and is responsible for the "rapid rush" that many long-distance runners experience.

When you're ready, please focus on giving yourself the following reminder message: "Out of a world of infinite possibilities, I am free in every new moment to choose what I focus my thoughts and feelings on and, as a consequence, the chemicals they secrete and the new experiences they bring into in my life."

You may be thinking, "That may be true, but what happens if I find myself running emotionally amuck creating a really bad day?" If that happens, immediately tell yourself, "Okay. It's time I take a hard look at what I'm focusing on, because

I'm the one who chooses how I feel and how I feel directs energy to attract matching future events.

I need to realize it's me who consciously creates my own destiny by my choice of thoughts and feelings."

If you make it a "bad" day—one you have formed by your thoughts and feelings, then ask yourself this next series of evocative questions:

1. Am I relinquishing my power as a conscious creator by choosing thoughts that generate bad-feeling chemicals?
2. Am I addicted to bad-feeling chemicals or good-feeling chemicals?
3. Am I in the habit of changing my focus and the chemicals they create the very moment I begin to feel bad?
4. Do I understand I may be addicted to bad emotions (molecules of feelings) from my past?

As you ponder these questions, begin focusing your attention on feeling-good thoughts. If you find it difficult to resist focusing on seemingly insurmountable obstacles, say to yourself, "I'm simply not thinking big enough. I'm not moving beyond my tiresome self-limiting beliefs. As the thinker of my thoughts, I have the built-in power to seize control and direct the energy of my thoughts in whichever direction I choose."

Recognize you use only those perceptions that give your preconceived beliefs, thoughts and feelings validity.

Creating a major mental shift in your health, relationships, job, whatever, is dependent on how you *think and feel*—the two most valuable assets in your life. If your private perspective is riddled with toxic and self-limiting thoughts, beliefs, expectations and feelings, you need to remind yourself how debilitating such an attitude can be. Whenever it occurs to you that you're *not* going to get through a particular crisis, the chemical messengers formed by your thoughts and feelings are sent from the brain to your cells, fostering an unhealthy environment that is likely to exacerbate the crisis, rather than alleviate it. Until you succeed in making that mental shift toward positive imagery I described a moment ago, your same old predictable dilemmas are likely to return to you time and time again.

My personal short and simple recommendation: Think of each repeated toxic thought and feeling as a chemical, not unlike having an addiction to a deadly street drug! To get yourself out of this self-defeating cycle you must stretch your conscious limits and keep reminding yourself that "like attracts like."

Your feelings reflect moment-by-moment exactly what you're thinking.

This being true, tell yourself, "For the next seven days, I'm going to change to new thoughts that will allow me to feel differently. No longer will I resist or deny that, as a conscious co-creator, I can conquer this crisis. I will simply think, feel, and know inwardly that the outcome I want to bring into my life has already happened in this present moment."

Does that message feel good? Does it feel like you're heeding the messages of your inner voice—your link to the authority of your soul? If so, then go with it.

Ready for another "Eureka" moment? Here it is: Let's say you're suddenly introduced to new healthier ways of thinking

144

which affect your physical well-being and attract healthier events into your life—by reading this book, for example. You may find, sadly, that these healthy new thoughts are unable to break into the rigid thought patterns you've created because of your addiction to past feelings. Until you do succeed in breaking old patterns, you'll continue to experience more of the same old same old. For new healthy thoughts to work, you need to get habituated to them.

Chemicals are feelings and feelings are chemicals.

What makes this back-to-wellness process a hindrance is that the new healthier thoughts you've been introduced to have not yet formed new feelings (new healthy chemical messengers). That will not happen until you begin perceiving them as *real*. Only then will the cells in your body feel and quickly react to the molecular messages that you're sending. If you fail to emphatically envision a new state of affairs as being real, the changes you desire will not take place.

This is why, when you tell yourself (or others tell you), "There's no possible way I can do that!", you need to counter with, "Oh, yes I can!" simply because you are what you think and feel!

The daily practice of outcome-oriented visualization to supplant and eradicate damaging thoughts and feelings will allow you to begin producing the positive feelings that will make growth and healing possible. After all, you're on this planet to learn about creating yourself and gaining wisdom from each experience you encounter.

No one ever fails Life 101. You're here to learn. And if you don't get it—whatever it is you're meant to learn—you're going to keep getting it until you get it.

One of the richest joys in life comes from understanding that you're playing by the rules (beliefs, expectations and feelings) you yourself make. The challenge lies in successfully forming these new habits of mind. How can you bring this about? Start by smiling with your mouth and eyes, then begin visualizing with emotion the outcome you want to achieve as a completed event. Next, envision the outpouring of serotonin and norepinephrine, while telling yourself: "Nothing on earth is more important than my creating good-feeling thoughts, since that's what I'll attract into my life."

Now do you "get" why it's so important to mentally stay in a good-feeling place? If chaos theory is correct and chaos creates eventual change that *strengthens* a system, it's critical to monitor your thoughts and feelings so each thought and feeling vibration attracts joyful vibrations that you want to enter your life.

By your perceptions YOU form physical reality as you know it!

What you should be telling yourself right about now is, *"Whatever I have created, I can un-create, at any present time I choose."*

But you need to be certain what you want and what you think and feel are in vibrational alignment. For example, saying, "I think I can get through this crisis, but I'm not really sure I can make it happen," is *not* a vibrational match-up. However, stating, "I know I'll get through this situation, because I see and feel it as having already happened," does coincide exactly with what you think, feel and want, and is in vibrational alignment. It's a matter of sustaining the vibrant and positive thrust of your thought, rather than allowing the insidious mist of negativity to creep in and undermine its power and focus.

More advice to ponder: Be aware how a particular situation feels to you and, right off the bat, you'll know what chemicals are flowing through your bloodstream—sometimes even before the matching event it attracts can enter your life.

As I've stated many times,

YOU create the external world you internally inhabit. Therefore, the answers you're looking for are not "out there." They're within!

Have you ever been entranced by a gaggle of geese flying V-like in almost perfect formation high overhead? Ever notice how suddenly, the entire flock will change directions, almost simultaneously? Does the leader send a signal to each bird individually? There is no time for that. Rather, they are collectively communicating, focused on the same frequency by means of a little-understood process that biologists call entrainment. We would say that all the geese are *operating on the same wave length*. Much the same thing occurs when you place a baby adjacent to its mother's breast. The baby and the mother's heart beat will beat rhythmically together.

Here are a few more examples of entrainment. If you find yourself agreeing with someone on a topic that you feel quite strongly about and hook up both your brains to an oscilloscope, you'll find brain wave patterns that coincide. People in love exhibit the same brain patterns. If you start clocks with a pendulum swinging at different times, eventually they'll begin swinging in unison. Women in prison often have the same menstrual cycles.

Deepak Chopra has pointed out that if you take a group of mice and give them an electric shock, remove them from the room and bring other mice in, as soon as the new mice enter the room, they panic. Know why? They inhale the hormones of fear produced by the other mice. There is reason to believe this happens in humans as well. What these examples suggest is that we're all connected vibrationally.

Have you ever (a) entered a room and felt anxious; (b) been to a memorial when you can actually feel the vibrations running up and down your spine; (c) been to a sacred place and felt a sense of calmness and loving compassion; (d) met someone and within seconds, think that this person seems a bit off-center, out of tune? The point is that it's through thought and feeling we communicate.

What thoughts and feelings are you entraining with? For example, do you think and feel that you're on the same frequency with what you really want in life? Ask yourself, "Am I open-minded enough to embrace new thoughts that allow me to move ahead by leaps and bounds?" "Am I willing to change old, obsolete, non-working thoughts that are not working for me, or do I cling to thoughts and feelings I should leave behind me?" "Do I have a job that brings meaning into my life?"

Nietzsche once said, "He who has a why to live can bear with any how." Think of his statement this way: People who have a reason and purpose to live can meet life head-on and consistently co-create the future experiences they want to enter their lives. The reason is we're all a part of Universal Consciousness. We're all connected. Because we live in a holographic universe, each of us mirrors the whole. We're all one.

Universal Consciousness is a sea of quantum soup—a field of unlimited energy—an energy field of all possibilities out of which we can create what we choose. We have limitless choices at our disposal because we too are a field of infinite possibilities. "We are," said Jane Roberts, "inside God. We are "literally made of God-stuff and we are eternal." So right about now you should be asking yourself: "Maybe I ought to stop and think what would happen in my life if I started thinking beyond my current self-limiting beliefs—started thinking without limits."

Now, even though it's not my personal responsibility, let me ask you this critical question:

When *specifically* (time and date) are you planning to alter the state of your current fate by changing any toxic and off-kilter thoughts and feelings you presently are focusing attention upon?

You have to start the *toxic thoughtectomy* process somewhere. So why not, right now, break free from self-sabotaging thoughts and feelings and start developing the authentic power that is inherently yours as a conscious co-creator?

Getting back to my bottom-line question: "When *specifically* are you planning to change the state of your current fate by changing your toxic beliefs and thoughts?" As an aside, do you happen to remember Newton's Third Law of Motion? It says, "A body in motion stays in motion, while a body at rest…" If you didn't get what I'm getting at, the subject is:

Inertia, revisited!

We're talking about live negative energy with absolutely no liberating potential to create peace of mind. For rarely does inertia "sow an act and reap a benefit," especially physical and spiritual well-being. Nor does it "sow a character and reap a beneficial destiny." That's why, to energize your life, you need to keep the momentum (i.e. the flow of positive vibrating energy) going and going and going, just like the bunny in the Energizer Battery commercial. This action is called

Purposeful determination.

Purposeful determination is persistently flowing positive energy. It's knowing that each of us is a conscious co-creator, not just a reactor to life's blend of dramatic self-created plots. It's being aware of how quick you need to be in altering your toxic focus, so you can allow your *wants* to enter your life.

Perhaps now is the opportune moment to upgrade your life by seeking out the hidden patterns and rules that you live by, which may be at odds with your deepest values.

Intention is the trigger to change. Your thoughts invest your feelings with energy via your intent (i.e., strong desire). As Reverend Shuller said, "If it's going to be, it's up to me." He was right on target as well when he said, "Inch by inch, anything's a cinch."

As a cancer survivor, I'll tell you a heavy lesson I learned: It's that often what appears to be an end, in essence is a new beginning. Of course, that's true only if you choose to perceive yourself as a "taboo-breaker"—one who wants to stay in resonance with cosmic vibrations. And, according to author and professor of psychology Sonja Lyubomirsky, Ph.D., those vibrating feelings will spur the striving to set more goals in an upward spiral. You may also want to listen to the advice of author Edward Teller: "When you get to the end of all the light you know," he said, "and it's time to step into the darkness of the unknown, faith is knowing that one of two things shall happen; either you will be given something solid to stand on, or you will be taught to fly."

A new, intense, positive thought and feeling is far more powerful than an existing negative event that already is present in your life.

To help you get the momentum of wellness energy started, it's suggested you read and sign the *Soul Agreement* in Appendix I. It's For Your Eyes Only.

Chapter Eleven

NEVER SAY DIE
Universal Consciousness:
The Creative Energy Essence Behind
Beliefs and Emotions that Form Your Life
Experiences

*"Consciousness is that by which this world first
becomes manifest."*

– Erwin Shrodinger,
quantum physicist and Nobel Laureate

The surrounding energy of Universal or God Consciousness represents a limitless field of future possibilities that, according to quantum physics, become "real(ity)" only when observed or focused upon by conscious beings. Drawing daily from its limitless field of creative energy, your focused thoughts and feelings cause matching physical likenesses to appear in your life.

Because you may not be familiar with the terminology I'm using here, it may be worthwhile to point out that the energy field of Universal or God Consciousness can also be termed ALL THAT IS, Infinite Energy, Holy Spirit, Adonai, Universal Mind, Source Energy, Ultimate Reality, Infinite Power, Intelligent Energy, Higher Self, Pure Awareness, Creative Mind, Brahman, and so on.

The reason a familiarity with these concepts is so crucial to spiritual development is that you are not distinct from, but a part of them. You are a part of Universal Consciousness, which is within you. You are by birth individualized consciousness—a *co-creator*.

Think of it this way: The kingdom of Universal or God consciousness is implanted within each of us. It is the "very process itself," says author Ken Wilber in *A Brief History of Everything*. The big, hard question we're addressing here is Why you, or anyone else, would deliberately give up this power in order to advance the opposite position—that of a powerless victim? You've been given a conscious mind, and through concentrated focus, you can direct your energies toward giving birth to constructive beliefs, thoughts, and expectations. These positive imaginings, in turn, tend to facilitate precisely the beliefs and expectations they contain. As the philosopher Sun Tzu once observed, "Opportunities multiply as they are seized."

Gregg Bradden, in his paradigm-shattering book, *The Divine Matrix*, states, "Experimental evidence is leading to a conclusion that we're actually creating the universe as we go and adding to what already exists! In other words, we appear to be the very energy that's forming the cosmos, as well as the beings who experience what we're creating."

Nobel Prize winner and quantum physicist John Wheeler is suggesting we live in a "participatory universe." In his own words, Wheeler says, "we could not even imagine a universe that did not somewhere and for some stretch of time contain observers, because the very building materials of the universe are these acts of observer-participancy." That is to say, since we live in an observer-created, thought-responsive universe, there is no reality until it is perceived reality.

Once you accept that consciousness (the sum of your beliefs and expectations) creates the material world—that nothing exists until someone observes or focuses on it, you need to ask yourself this question: "On a daily basis what am I choosing to focus consciousness on? Is it the present, the past, or am I mostly delegating power to worries about the future?"

The present moment is the only point where creative, life-changing events take place. If you fail to enter and dwell in that domain, you will be undermining your innate ability as a conscious co-creator to significantly reverse the negative aspects of your life. "The distinction between past, present, and future is only a stubbornly persistent illusion," said Albert Einstein. "Time," he said, "is not at all what it seems. It does not flow in only one direction, and the future exists simultaneously with the past."

When people heal themselves, they have consciously said, "Enough already!" They have rejected an illness and inserted in the present moment a new future probability into their past, where no physical problem, a healthy probability, existed. The critical elements: the focused belief and expectation of already achieving wellness, and the inner knowledge of your own power to allow your limitless soul—an unending universal energy field that houses your physical body—the freedom to soar in time and space.

Here's more counsel for advanced souls: Have you ever wondered why you're on this planet? The short answer is that you are meant to learn how to gain life-transforming knowledge and skill in manipulating and managing the energy of your thoughts and emotions. That skill involves paying careful attention to how your thoughts form matching physical experiences, and becoming aware that the moment you focus on past wounds and hurts, you re-create and re-traumatize the past as present "facts." Most of all it involves setting your objectives clearly and plainly and then becoming one with them. It's thinking, believing, and feeling, from a position of completion, as if results were already present "facts." As Thomas Paine advises in *Common Sense*: "A long habit of not thinking something wrong gives it a superficial appearance of being right."

You are a "spiritual work in progress"—an evolving consciousness in physical form in a training process for developing consciousnesses. It's not waiting someday to see what fate has in store for you. It's seizing the "someday" in this present moment! You learn and evolve spiritually through the successful and failed realities you create.

It won't do to tell yourself, "I'll *try* changing my toxic beliefs and feelings." You must make a "can-do" commitment to stick with this book's "Back-to-Wellness Program." The projected outcome: The reachable goal of wellness in virtually all areas of your life—psychologically, emotionally and physically. As William R. Lucas said, "That which you vividly imagine, sincerely believe, ardently desire, and enthusiastically act upon, will inevitably come to pass." That being said, are you thinking? "That which is like unto itself is drawn." Excellent. That's the overall rule of thumb to keep in mind.

One prerequisite to charting a back-to-wellness course successfully is to recognize and acknowledge that supercharging your health and life will require constant effort. It's a simple matter of **use versus disuse**. Scientific studies on how the brain functions suggest that neural pathways require repeated use to survive. Through daily practice you will succeed in creating new neural pathways to bolster your new and positive mental outlook. But without such continued effort, no real transformation is likely to take place.

Please Note:

Information will be repeated here that has been stated before. There is a reason: To help you derive optimum benefit from the simple principle I am advancing, that you have the inherent ability to consciously create the life events you want to experience. But why take my word for it? If you put the exercises in Appendix II into practice you'll see for yourself how effective your Inner Senses are in giving birth to your physical world.

The question arises: What should I do if I get a grim diagnosis or lab test and start thinking, "I just know I'm not going to make it!"

The answer: Recognize that you perceive life through the filter of personal beliefs, thoughts, feelings, and expectations that actually *form* the world you experience. In other words, you get what you perceive. If you focus on the self-limiting belief, "I just know I'm not going to make it," this belief makes a probable outcome of wellness highly unlikely.

Your beliefs and feelings can increase or diminish wellness inasmuch as they direct the health of your cells. Your thought, "I just know I'm not going to make it!" is a self-sabotaging obstruction to wellness, because life can't give you wellness unless you succeed in forcefully allowing its future probability into your belief system. That's why it's so important for you to ask yourself, "What lens (set of beliefs) am I viewing life through? Is it illness or wellness?

In previous chapters I have outlined several simple principles that will help you to stop false and harmful beliefs. The first is…

Your inner Self (psyche, soul, consciousness) is NOT limited.

As an individualized part of Universal Consciousness (i.e., God Consciousness, Divine Spirit, Holy Spirit) you are a spiritual being in a physical body having a human experience. Your individualized Self or consciousness exists with eternal authenticity, and as such it has no limitations. To deny the importance of each individual consciousness is to deny the importance of Universal Consciousness for the two exist one within the other. You (individualized consciousness) and Universal consciousness are inseparable. Each person is an aspect of Universal Consciousness.

Ours is an unfinished world, one in a state of becoming, waiting for human beings to continue the work of Universal Consciousness. Since Universal Consciousness is unlimited, limitations that you experience are the result of limiting beliefs, thoughts and feelings that you have deliberately chosen to accept, which take the form of life experiences. You are accountable for your life because you choose which life events you want to materialize. For example, if you think and feel, "I'm not going to make it!" you'll search out only those "facts" that tend to back up your toxic belief.

I learned a second principle to help prevent limiting beliefs from emerging while studying quantum physics and interviewing long-term cancer survivors who had defied and grown beyond the grim prognoses given to them by the scientific community.

YOU are a "Reality Co-creator" (a divine gift). YOU form your own life experiences (or they're formed for you)!

To understand this fundamental principle, you need to move out of a "group think" mentality and learn to experience yourself as separate from your *beliefs* about yourself. Scrutinize your core beliefs as you would a painting you've created and are now standing back from. If you're not pleased with it, then consciously and with strong intent and feeling, change the painting (mental pictures) in your mind by daily practice of the "Back-to-Wellness" tools you'll find in Appendix II. These back-to-wellness strategies will help you identify and unlearn your limiting beliefs, which will allow you to reclaim your power as a conscious co-creator.

The big "AHA" you'll observe over time is this: What you firmly believe, think, expect and feel will emerge in physical form as life experiences! The task at hand is to visualize healthy beliefs, thoughts and feelings as already finished future events!

As a co-creator of your life events, your imagination and feelings are the most concentrated forms of energy you possess. They form your ideas of yourself and the world as you perceive it. They direct your very existence!

Outcome-oriented imagery combined with strong belief, feelings, and intent, project thoughts in the form of energy from your inner Self to your body and to the physical world, constantly shaping and forming your creations. In fact, your thoughts and feelings are electromagnetic energy (atoms and molecules) in motion, which move through space and time. Not only do they affect your physical body but also the physical conditions surrounding you.

Consider the highly complex nature of your body purely from the physical standpoint. You perceive your body as solid mass, as you perceive all matter; yet in fact we might say with equal accuracy that within your body, energy takes on specific shapes in the form of cells, molecules, atoms and electrons, each combining to form matter. The body that appears so solid turns out to be composed of rapidly moving particles, often circling each other, in which vast transfers of energy continually occur. Again,

You are in a training ground for transforming the energy of your beliefs, thoughts, and feelings into valuable life experiences.

Be mindful that any damaging belief you accept as "truth" is a potential experience you yourself have chosen. I am suggesting that you remind yourself that, "This erroneous belief isn't necessarily true, even though I *believe* it." You must learn to disregard all beliefs that in any way limit you as a conscious co-creator.

On the next page you'll find a list of common self-limiting beliefs, thoughts and feelings. If you find yourself agreeing with any of these expressions, you have steered off the "Back-to-Wellness" course. Remember that:

YOU bring your beliefs, thoughts and feelings alive. A negative belief you think today, unless changed, will be experienced tomorrow!

The list on the next page will short-cut your education by helping you more fully appreciate how the power of fear, encoded in belief and thought, can contribute to the bleak consequences that images and feelings of victimization invite. The physical body can defend against illness but not the sustained fear of illness.

Pessimistic and fearful mental programming can be a drag on the functioning of your immune system, leading to a lifetime of poor health. If you find yourself identifying with one or more of the toxic beliefs listed in the box on the next page, ask yourself, "What probable future outcome is this belief I'm focusing on already attracting into my life?"

1. I just know I'm not going to make it!
2. I'm helpless before circumstances I just can't control.
3. I'm helpless because my character was formed at an early age and I'm totally at the mercy of my past.
4. I have the same symptoms Mary had, and she's gone you know.
5. A rare cure sometimes happens in others but it's not likely to ever happen to me.
6. Things can only go down hill from here.
7. No matter how hard I try, I'm never going to make it. Any way you look at it, it's just not in the cards.
8. I always see a worse case scenario. I can't help myself, that's who I am.
9. When it rains it pours.
10. I'm losing my energy. It's not what it used to be.
11. I can't seem to see and hear as well as I used to.
12. Everything that happens to me is fate. If it's meant to be, it's meant to be.
13. Bad news from the CT scan, I won't make it.
14. If I hear any bad news, I come unglued.
15. This is just not my day.
16. Cancer (heart attacks, etc.) run in my family. The way things are going in my life, I'm probably next.
17. I'll grow sicker and lose my mental powers as I grow old.
18. When my body dies, my consciousness passes away with it.
19. I've always been a bit pessimistic. I'll probably never change.

Individuals who focus on the core beliefs listed above are attracting to themselves a corresponding probable future reality. Your effective power to move back to wellness will be sapped by such thoughts and feelings, which also sustain the inner reality that feeds your illness. The issues behind illness often contain challenges meant to lead you to greater spiritual growth, but you won't be able to meet those challenges if your energies are bound up in toxic thinking. The life lesson: ***What you think and feel—you experience!***

Unfortunately the path back to wellness is seldom easy to find on your own. It has taken me over a decade of research, personally interviewing long-term cancer survivors, conducting workshops on the subject, and making many mistakes, before developing the "Back-to-Wellness" program I am offering here. The fruits of my labors will free you of months of tiresome and problematic efforts covering the same ground. Practice the Quiet Miracles "Back-to-Wellness" Program and it will change your life forever! I wish that such a step-by-step guide had been available when I was diagnosed with cancer many years ago.

You get in life what you focus your attention on! Through your thoughts and fellings, YOU form your own internal and external experiences!

All well and good, you reply. But what happens if you find yourself in a vicious spiral in which you find yourself constantly painting pictures in your mind that reinforce the negative aspects in your life? In that case, I suggest that you take the following "break-the-glass-in-case-of-emergency" actions:

(a) Make a clear distinction between you and your beliefs—the rules you live by.

(b) Realize that your beliefs are physically formed.

(c) Understand that what you believe to be true in life is true.

(d) Take note that, to change a physical effect, you must change the original belief while recognizing that, for an interval of time, physical realization of the old beliefs may still be part of your "reality."

(e) Have confidence that your new beliefs will quickly begin to show themselves in your life as actual experiences.

And here is another perfectly healthy suggestion. Playfully visualize a game where you adopt a belief , for example, "Every day in every way I know I AM getting healthier and healthier!" that you strongly desire to see as "fact." (In the chapters to come you will find the Outcome-Oriented Visualization Technique, The Suspension of Damaging Thoughts Technique, and The Prayer Dream Technique, to help you.) Imagine what you picture happening in your mind as an existing reality. Know that all events are mental and psychic first and that these will become probable future events, but don't keep watching yourself. Know and expect that you'll experience in your life what you believe and mentally envision. Also, continue to preface your affirmations by saying, "I KNOW," which is far more powerful an intention than "I believe." For example, say to yourself, "I KNOW that every day in every way I AM perfectly healthy." Cultivating an inner sense of KNOWING is a very simple tactic that stops self-limiting beliefs, since it is unlimited in scope.

Since all knowledge resides within and not without, by requesting before you fall asleep (See Prayer/Dream Exercise in Appendix II) that answers to problems be given to you when you awaken, you instinctively begin seeding and tapping into your dream knowledge to a far greater extent. Remember: Even in the dream state, what you focus attention on, you experience!

What if you were to say to me, "I really could care less about your wellness strategies. My case is totally different. Statistics show that people with my illness simply don't make it"?

I would reply that statistics simply do NOT apply to individuals. I would also remind you that all thoughts are energy in motion. Thus, jumping to a "worse-case conclusion" (via a negative mental filter), by the very nature of its intense focus, will propel you into an accelerated self-fulfilling creation of powerlessness. The consequences of such pessimistic mental programming on suppressing your immune system can be very detrimental.

Since "like attracts like," your first action is to identify and quickly change your negative self-talk (toxic energy). Here's why:

Your cells are listening to and carrying out your instructions (self-talk) in a loyal manner.

Think about it: You can't lack confidence in your own capacity to get back to wellness, and at the same time believe in the unlimited nature of Universal Consciousness. This is because Universal Consciousness is the creative source energy of your physical being. As a portion of Universal Consciousness, if your essential nature is imperfect, so must be that of Universal Consciousness.

Consider this option: Chart your self-talk and your focus of thought and expectation daily. If you find yourself unable to shake the belief that the universe is merely a batch of atoms and molecules that have randomly been energized into consciousness, then you will find it difficult to accept that you have conscious control over your destiny. On the contrary, it will seem that you are powerless. With such thoughts in mind, a debilitating biochemical reality is likely to follow that will inhibit and undercut the very mental immunity you're searching for.

Begin *attacking* and *separating* yourself from your toxic beliefs, since any belief you constantly strengthen is likely to create the matching environment in your body and a corresponding future event.

You may think and believe, "Every day in every way, I know I AM perfectly healthy. This is my new belief." Yet conditions remain the same. So you think, "My conscious thoughts simply aren't working to create what I believe." You can not have conflicting thoughts and feelings and expect to experience what you strongly desire. Incidentally, you may want to look to those areas of your life that are successful. You'll see the same belief mechanisms at work.

A shortcut to stop negative thoughts that works for me and can work for you.

When faced with the situation described above, I demand from myself that I stop a harmful belief by picturing a stop sign followed by the expressed affirmation "Every day, in every way, I know I am perfectly healthy." I then proceed to act as if this is true. Sometimes, I'll actually yell and scream STOP! at a toxic belief I find myself focusing on. After yelling (when I am alone, of course) at a damaging belief or thought, I then forget about it, trusting and knowing inwardly that my new belief will change the negative circumstances in my life.

Your cells believe every word you tell them and respond obediently! Remind yourself that your cells rely on your personal interpretation of the environment and react in precise biological conformity to your expectations.

The emotional condition of many patients is so vulnerable that they readily accept declarations made under seemingly dire circumstances by healthcare professionals. As a result, the patient may feel relatively hopeless and helpless, and at the mercy of both the illness and the scientific community. Remaining in this highly focused "trance state," not unlike a subject who is given suggestions by a hypnotist, the patient unwittingly accepts the negative suggestions, not suspecting that every cell in his or her body is listening to and faithfully following these personal instructions. Since energy flows where attention goes, it's evident that you can't get well as long as you continue to believe and feel you can't.

As a portion of Universal Consciousness you are meant to evolve spiritually by widening your spectrum of life experiences!

World-wide research conducted on out-of-body (OOB) and near-death-experiences (NDEs) merely confirms what anecdotal evidence accumulated over centuries has suggested—that human consciousness (the psyche or soul) is eternal and has a sacred right to life. In the deepest sense, there is no death. All that exists is a change of focus by individual consciousness, which has left physical reality. Consciousness then moves about freely in another dimension. In actuality, we achieve this state each night in the dream environment. Like the dream state, the after-death environment is simply one in which different laws apply. Both states are far less limiting than the physical reality in which we daily operate.

You experiment with probable future life experiences while in the dream state.

In either the awake or dream state, each of us is a conscious co-creator of our life experiences! An excellent wellness technique I practice is to awaken each morning acknowledging that I have at my command limitless life choices to form my day. I remind myself that I'm a conscious co-creator, capable of transforming my thoughts and expectations into probable future life events. What returning to wellness is all about, after all, is constructively thinking of each day as a blank slate and asking yourself, "What future outcome am I going to form on that slate today?" The reason: Every thought (pulsating energy) you have accepted as "fact" has a dictated result. The same kind of thought habitually repeated will be perceived to have a permanent effect. Awareness of your present thoughts can be used to check your physical and spiritual progress. If you don't like what you're experiencing (e.g. illness, relationship issues, financial or job challenges, etc.) you must change your conscious thoughts and expectations. Otherwise you can not become the person (soul) you're meant to be.

Quantum physics is suggesting that structure follows expectation and that matter, at any time, can be altered by the activation of the creative factors inherent in all consciousness.

What existence comes down to is taking an ontological approach to life. As you become more fully aware of your own being, your self-talk, and your own central beliefs, it may be easier to acknowledge that you have the power to change your inner thoughts and expectations, "knowing" all the while that your outer environment will change accordingly. "Destiny," said William Jennings Bryant, "is not a matter of chance, it is a matter of choice; it is not a thing to be waited for, it is a thing to be achieved."

Since you form the future with your every thought, an existential shift or dramatic change in personal belief and thought will be required to create a beneficial set of life circumstances. This being the case, why not try a thought experiment for seven days, practicing the notion that "You get in life what you focus your attention on!" It could become a life experiment.

The idea is to think of yourself as a living laboratory, knowing that any belief you constantly reinforce is likely to form a matching outer experience. Under this creative thought experiment, you'll see for yourself—you become the self you think you are. *You are what you think about!* Practicing this thought experiment will condition you to think of yourself as a perfectly healthy person. Simply keep reminding yourself that, "I am Individualized Consciousness, a portion of Universal Consciousness, and therefore unlimited." This powerful affirmation can go a long way to help you expand your definition of what's possible in life. Since you are individualized consciousness and a vital force in the universe, why not begin right now to stop perpetuating illness and instead create wellness? I say "right now", because *the creative present moment is your maximum position of power!*

Indeed, if every thought is a future event, think of how powerful you really are in this present moment of creation.

Since quantum physics is suggesting that past, present and future exist simultaneously, by staying in the present moment with your every thought, you quite factually can create new healthier life experiences. The new science also suggests that you can change your present condition by reprogramming your past. It all follows from focusing intently on the present moment. This is because every probable YOU exists and is active in the field of probabilities. It is solely your responsibility via conscious choice to determine which "future you" or "future event" you choose to bring into your life. With your every thought, your life can take any turn you fully believe, feel and picture as physically realized. To that extent, anyway you look at life,

Believing is seeing!

In this existence as a co-creator, you are learning to handle the inexhaustible energy that is at all times available to you. What is necessary is to become totally immersed in the present moment of creation, free of all past or present harmful thoughts and expectations, such as anger, resentment, and past wounds. Disagreements in relationships, for example, often arise when you choose to transfer ownership of your inherent power as a co-creator to someone else. Once you regain your powerful role as a co-creator of your own experiences, there is not a soul on earth who can make you angry or fearful, since you alone choose the products of your creation. From this point of view, you can not help being self-directed and self-responsible. Knowing you're a part of Universal Consciousness, you'll recognize that it is possible to change the outcome of an event before it enters your life as an experience.

Isn't it about time you reclaimed your power as a conscious co-creator?

The strength and duration of a life event is dependent on the intent and intensity of the thoughts and feelings that generate it. You can achieve your personal goals through the "Back-to-Wellness Action Plan" by daily combining strong belief, thought, feeling, and outcome-oriented imagery, forming them into a mental picture of the physical effects you strongly desire. Be assured that having the courage of your convictions and taking forward action will give you an opportunity to experience a more profound and higher level of consciousness.

It should be emphasized that starting and sticking to the "Back-to-Wellness Action Plan" is solely up to you. Eleanor Roosevelt summed up the situation you face when she said, "You must do the things that you cannot do—you get strength, courage, and confidence by every experience in which you really stop to look fear in the face."

Chapter 12

End Fear and Stress Right NOW!

"The only thing we have to fear is fear itself, nameless unreasoning, unjustified terror which paralyses needed efforts to convert retreat into advance."

– Franklin D. Roosevelt

B onding with media health announcements can be hazardous to your health.

Have you noticed the recent proliferation of public health announcements (and pharmaceutical ads) on radio, television, newspapers, billboards, popular publications, and countless other outlets, warning us about various dangers to our health?

"Do you have the following 7 symptoms of breast cancer ..."

"New tests to look for if you have prostate cancer .... "

"Do you have hidden heart disease? Here's how to know:"

"Five signs of severe depression."

"Memory Loss? Here's what to watch for!"

"Tired? Discover your tiredness profile."

"Here's a checklist to see if you have hypertension:"

"Here's how to know if you have diabetes:"

These salvos of medical advice may be well-intentioned, but I can assure you that their effect on consumers who are highly prone to suggestion can be devastating. In fact, such warnings and advice often feed our fears, and can actually form the physical symptoms they're describing.

Think about it: Each time you're asked to examine yourself for a specific bodily symptom—even though you may currently feel healthy—in effect, you are putting yourself in the same position as those highly suggestive medical students we spoke about earlier, who take on the generalized symptoms of the diseases they're studying. Here's what happens: (a) You focus on the image of a specific symptom. (b) The subconscious, through the Law of Attraction, sets the mental picture into operation. (c) The symptom begins to manifest itself in the body. Is it not ironic that physicians who succumb to this process as students often underestimate, in their later practice, the enormous influence their suggestive declarations (beliefs) have to highly impressionable patients? Sadly, once a disabling belief is accepted and transferred, it becomes embedded in the subconscious mind and actualized to fruition. Many lose sight of the fact that abnormal cell formation can be increased as well as decreased by highly intense beliefs and emotions.

Why it is the American public so often focuses on illness and not wellness?

Some long-term cancer survivors working with the power of suggestion (natural hypnosis) bring about remarkably restorative changes in their minds and bodies. Conversely, the power of suggestion, if graphically and acutely presented, can just as remarkably prepare the mind to work against itself, in precisely the manner described above. The result?

A blueprint for illness:

The repetitive power of public and commercial health messages such as, "Do you have the following seven symptoms of breast cancer?" are stomach churners that feed vividly into the public's most dreaded fears. When repeated often enough, such messages can, via negative mental imagery, suggestively advance the illness being portrayed. Drawn by fear, and open and receptive to the suggestions of others, impressionable listeners and viewers fail to realize that they have created these emerging physical symptoms (which they accept as true and inevitable) themselves, under the powerful influence of these frequent public health messages. In short, they get exactly what they are looking for.

Today's entire health prevention industry is administering a relentless placebos-like message, and it's proving to be remarkably effective. But in their health announcements, it isn't doctors, but actors or celebrities garbed in white coats, with stethoscopes hanging around their necks, who are doing the talking. I have a keen sense that, as a result of this highly profiled mental imagery, countless numbers of easily swayed listeners and viewers attract to themselves the dreaded symptoms they are cautioned to "watch out for." In a large measure, this is the placebo effect, magnified through the hidden force of repeated suggestion. Focusing on symptoms is certainly no way to maintain good health or get a new lease on life, especially if the chronic illness described is already dragging you down.

Fearful thoughts and feelings are toxic energy in motion. They magnetically attract illness. You then witness the illness your thoughts and feelings have formed. This provides "absolute evidence" for the "truth" of your toxic thoughts and feelings, a self-created loop of cause-and-effect that continues until you alter the source of your illness, your toxic thoughts and feelings.

All of us look at life through the eyes of our accepted beliefs. We act as if they exist as fundamental "truths." Fearful beliefs and thoughts are not truths. They are representations of your imagination and emotional interpretations. yet they dictate your life experiences. They can be translations of childhood fears, past wounds, or resentments you believe, nourish, and keep alive.

Such fearful beliefs narrow your path to wellness. They can cause disease. It is therefore critical to identify and supplant these invisible beliefs, thoughts and expectations that trigger feelings of fear with supportive beliefs.

Starting from where you are, positive beliefs are your access point, your door to move from fear to freedom.

The lesson to be learned is that you author the beliefs, thoughts, and feelings you live by. Why put limits on yourself? With proper techniques, you can re-script fear-based dominating beliefs and move to a position of self-empowerment. For example, let's say you choose to give energy to fear through the belief you are powerless to alter your medical condition, a relationship, job issues, and so on. This inhibiting belief gives rise to feelings of hopelessness—a strong emotional energy field that can strengthen the disease process. Interpret a particular life event through a kaleidoscope of fear-based images and the living pictures that develop are colored by your limiting beliefs. The emotions you experience, including fear, are a reflection of your inner reality.

What comes alive in your body and physical universe begins initially in your mind, in the form of healthy or unhealthy beliefs, thoughts and emotions. To alter the living picture of the world as you perceive it and to recover your sense of joy, it's important to remember what you experience inside, you experience outside.

172

It is equally relevant to realize that unresolved emotional problems can change your energy field and give rise to disease.

Your reality is formed by the intense energy of your thoughts and expectations. The more intense your fearful beliefs, thoughts, and self-talk, the sooner they develop in your physical body and as life experiences.

> *"Fears are educated into us and can, if we wish,*
> *be educated out,"*
> – Karl A. Menninger. MD.

For a rather lengthy period, I was asked to undergo cancer detection tests. During the first few appointments, I was quick to picture a worst-case scenario. Entrapped in the energy of fearful thoughts of doom and gloom, it was little wonder I experienced what I intensely focused attention on. Had I closely examined my most intimate thoughts and expectations, I would have known the reality I chose to create. Namely, more fear and anxiety. What I failed to perceive was that my experience originated in my ominous thoughts and expectations. My expectations were focused on the idea that things could only get worse. As a result of the intense belief I was powerless to change my medical condition, I found myself *feeling* that way. Focusing habitually on feelings of hopelessness totally convinced me that my beliefs were fundamentally true.

Belief is the "real" culprit!

Reminding myself that belief is the root that arouses and intensifies feelings forced me to realize that I myself had mentally generated the string of dreadful images I was experiencing. I also came to recognize that if I were to identify and monitor my destructive beliefs, I could replace them with new optimistic beliefs, and thereby unblock the necessary energy I needed to rid myself of the physical problem I was experiencing. A big moment of enlightenment occurred when I read a passage in my favorite book entitled, *The Nature of Personal Reality* by Jane Roberts. It stated that my beliefs belong to me but categorically are not me. That was an enormous eye-opener!

I was aware from my background in hypnosis that I needed to identify and replace my fearful beliefs and negative self-talk. I needed to acknowledge that I was stuck in a life role I myself had consciously chosen to structure. Reminding myself that I was a conscious co-creator and that it was possible to get unstuck and form new favorable beliefs took a great deal of internal hard work. "Still," I asked myself, "what was the downside?" The live feedback that my internal pessimism was reflecting in my mind, body and life was more than evident. In addition, I was totally convinced my beliefs, thoughts and expectations were realistic and could not be altered. Looking back, it's difficult for me to understand that, for me, my core belief in hopelessness was more *realistic* than a belief in hopefulness, even though this hopelessness was a subjective state formed by viewing life through the lens of a victim mentality. My highly toxic mental state reminded me to once again read Dr. Martin Seligman's book *Learned Optimism*—from cover to cover. At that moment, it was clear that my unbalanced mental attitude could easily have been titled, *Learned Pessimism*!

Ridding yourself of fear is an inside job

A piece of my mind still did not trust completely that I had uncovered an almost magical way to dematerialize fear from my life. As I continued to practice outcome-oriented visualization and the other wellness strategies disclosed in Appendix

II, it became more and more noticeable that change takes place from the "inside out." The life lesson: any way you perceive it, life truly is an "inside out" job.

To better my life, I was learning another necessary lesson:

To evolve to a higher level of consciousness, resistance perpetuates fear.

In those deeply blue periods when I was absolutely convinced I was about to die, I discovered that resistance creates even more fear. In *The Gift of Fear*, Gavin De Becker says, "The important question is not 'How might we die?', but rather, 'How shall we live?'" Besieged with the fear of dying, I learned that what you resist, persists and that "learned helplessness" most definitely needs to be ignored.

A simple exercise to give you peace and comfort.

Each night before falling asleep, for seven days prior to visiting my oncologist for cancer detection tests, I focused, with intense feelings, on practicing outcome-oriented visualization. Regardless of what my five senses were telling me, I visualized fear as a measly temporary condition. At the same time, I consciously incorporated into my wellness agenda an inner reality of highly optimistic self-talk. I made a personal commitment to myself to live completely in the present moment—in the Eternal Now. This prevented me from relapsing into past fearful mental images and the corresponding emotions that create "learned helplessness." Thinking of each new present moment that I had conquered as one in a series of successful present moments which would extend into hours, days and months, was for me, an epiphany.

To visualize the outcome of the cancer examination I strongly desired, here, in a nutshell, is what I consciously chose to emotionally imagine each night at bedtime, beginning one week prior to my oncology appointment:

(a) I "pictured" myself on the screen of my mind, entering the oncology clinic, breathing very slowly. I pictured my mind and body calm and at ease.

(b) Next, I "saw" myself taking the elevator to the doctor's office.

(c) In vivid detail, I then imagined progressing through the entire battery of tests in a completely relaxed mental and physical state.

(d) I completed each nightly session by giving myself a mental high five and saying "Yeah!" with a pumped fist. This punctuation added emotional intensity to each session, which I believe, hastened the outcome I strongly desired.

The accumulation and anchoring of these positive mental impressions—live, concentrated energy fields, coupled with the power of action—led to quite predictable results:

Seven days later, I completed the entire testing procedure virtually free of fear and anxiety.

By dissociating myself from my self-destructive beliefs, thoughts, and feelings, and forcefully attacking those beliefs, I succeeded in redirecting the vital energy they had consumed toward *restoring* my health and well-being. I moved from a sense of depression and powerlessness to a positive trait of "learned powerfulness" and the constructive emotions such an attitude generates. By changing my focus of attention, and reflecting on what could go *right* in my life, I used the same perceptive mechanisms that had fueled my pessimism, transforming a series of "no-can-do's" to mental impressions of "can-do's". And this moved me beyond the imprisonment of those toxic beliefs. The enriching lesson: You can't alter your life from the "outside in" when you live it "inside out!"

Changing your focus from a powerless position of fear, to confident self-empowerment, requires the following personal system of central beliefs and feelings:

* Being mentally receptive, opening your inner boundaries even to what you believe and emotionally feel is "not possible."
* Identifying your damaging beliefs, thoughts and feelings through self-assessment.
* Replacing the destructive beliefs you find with hopeful and beneficial ones.
* Positive self-talk, 24/7.
* Setting up favorable mental conditions so the subconscious can work for you—not against you.
* An unending awareness that you are a conscious co-creator and therefore have the inherent ability to visualize what you're capable of experiencing.
* Persistently remaining hopeful by picturing yourself on the screen of your mind with a fighting spirit.
* Continually pushing the boundaries of your limiting beliefs and thoughts.
* Repeatedly inducing an inward attitude of expectancy—and holding to that mental picture.
* Tuning each day into higher levels of awareness by asking for divine guidance to sense your soul's purpose.
* Making a conscious effort to attract a sense of joy and spontaneity into your life.

In reviewing *The Seth Material* by author Jane Roberts, from which numerous principles that I hold dear are derived, I found a wonderful exercise. The idea is to tell yourself

I will only respond to hopeful and helpful self-suggestions. This moment is now in the past. In this new present moment, I am already beginning to feel better and better." Then quickly focus your attention on something you thoroughly enjoy.

The sooner you use the exercises described in Appendix II to mitigate fear, the sooner you'll be able to cast off the toxic energy of fearful feelings that can precede or accompany virtually any crisis. You already have received an initiating course in "Beliefectomy 101" —the removal of toxic beliefs and fearful thoughts. Almost without knowing it, you've been introduced to its procedure. As you'll discover, releasing the toxic emotional energy of fear can have a clear-cut liberating influence for those who feel trapped by its disabling presence.

A brief background on how I got "here" (quieting my fearful emotions) from "there".

Specific physiological responses take place when we anticipate or find ourselves facing a profoundly frightening situation. Some or all of the following symptoms may become highly noticeable:

(a) shallow breathing

(b) perspiration

(c) increased blood pressure

(d) digestive problems

The following personal experience offers a case in point. After graduation from the University of Minnesota School of Pharmacy, I was working in a small retail pharmacy. At the time it was a fairly common occurrence to be robbed of narcotics at gunpoint. Strange as this may sound, I was not overcome with immobilizing fear while the robberies were in progress. It was the anticipation of a violent robbery I found terribly frightening. Compounding my anxiety was the fact that I seemed to have a knack for predicting in advance when a robbery would take place. In one instance, two strangers entered the pharmacy that I sensed were reconnoitering the premise. I could feel an almost immediate presence of an armed robbery set in on all levels of my being. My heart began to pound out of my chest. In such cases, my anxiety eventually triggered a migraine headache. Even when I was not at the pharmacy, the buildup of stress often reached the point where it affected my breathing.

How "real" were my physical disturbances? I'm embarrassed to recount the number of times I drove to the emergency room of a local hospital for EKG tests. With each visit, the physician in charge took me aside and said, "Look, you're just fine. Your symptoms appear to be the result of extreme stress due to the anticipation of an armed robbery."

To tone down my anxiety, I remember giving serious thought to asking my physician to prescribe a tranquilizer. Instead, I decided to try Transcendental Meditation which I found to be somewhat helpful. For some odd reason, I gave no thought to practicing visualization as an aid to managing the warning signs of robberies. My perceptions were situationally disposed in response to my anticipation of being robbed at gunpoint, or even perhaps getting killed, since very often robbers were "stoned" while in the act of committing a felony, or even worse. I could sense my inner voice telling me to honor who I was and to leave the job; that I was not a victim destined to live in fear. The message was clear: I had free will. I could alter my life script. As a conscious co-creator, I could look for ways to create a more beneficial set of experiences.

The question I confronted when anticipating an armed robbery at the pharmacy is really no different from the one faced by those who must deal with a life-threatening illness, "What am I going to do to alleviate the health-debilitating nature of fear?"

I took another step forward on my journey toward overcoming fear and cultivating a sense of well-being one day over lunch with Jim Peterson. A former NBA basketball player with the Houston Rockets, Jim is currently a TV announcer for the Minnesota Timberwolves. During the meal, he related a story about his guru, Paramanhasa Yogananda, one of the twentieth century's preeminent spiritual figures (a true bodhisattva, e.g., one who delays reaching nirvana in order to helps others), and the author of *Autobiography of a Yogi*. The book is a memorable "living teaching" that affords the reader a unique opportunity to gain a high degree of spiritual insight and understanding.

The Yogananda story Jim told me that day over lunch concerned a moment back in the thirties when the great yogi was seated in a movie theater pleasantly observing a series of scenes projected on a motion picture screen. Peering behind him, he could not help but notice a flickering beam of light streaming downward from the projection booth toward the dreamlike images unfolding on the screen below.

Using a picture show as a metaphor to represent the drama of life, and the projectionist in the booth of the cinema house as Divine Intelligence, Yogananda began to characterize life's conflicts and emotions in terms of the action and dialogue of a cosmic motion picture. He noted that the gateway to spiritual awakening and transformation is to recognize that everything in life is but a dream—an illusion—a figment of the five senses. (This concept is not unlike the one advanced by quantum physics that no experience is possible until there is an observer to perceive it.)

From a more universal vantage point, Yogananda began reflecting the many roles that humans play as spellbound participants on the screens of their minds. His conclusion: we should not take the fleeting film of existence so seriously, since the life drama we are dealing with is the illusory nature of Maya (cosmic delusion)—universal hypnosis. The following passage from Yogananda's book Autobiography of a Yogi expands on this simple concept:

> *Just as cinematic images that appear to be real are only combinations of light and shade, so is the universal variety a delusive seeming. The planetary spheres, with their countless forms of life, are naught but figures in a cosmic motion picture. Temporarily true to man's five sense perceptions, the transitory scenes are cast on the screen of human consciousness by the infinite creative beam.*

Staying with the calm before and after the storm.

Once I planted the picture show concept in my mind, I began to condition myself to believe Yogananda's simile could help me disconnect from the emotional energy of fear.

Yes, but would the idea of consciously changing my mental focus from a participant to a witness role in life's picture show actually work when I hit a sudden brick wall? Or, for that matter, when crisis became "deadly" serious?

With my newly formed thoughts and feelings, I realized I had found a way to consciously usher out fear's seemingly uncontrollable presence. As a conscious co-creator, I imagined I could self-create an extraordinarily deep wellness environment internally, which would form a like event externally. I reminded myself that reality appears to be in the circumstances that I presently am focusing attention on and, as a result, experiencing. I had to keep telling myself what's "real" is generated by the intensity of my thoughts and feelings, which I author internally and, as a consequence, experience externally. I reminded myself over and over again that nothing solid appears or is experienced until it's perceived. I decided to write the following on a Post-It™ note and paste in on my refrigerator door as a constant reminder: "What I think and feel is what I create." I underlined heavily, the word "I."

You are on this planet to learn essential life lessons.

At this time, I was achieving rapid progress in conquering my daily apprehensions by using the specific strategies discussed in Appendix II. Yet from time to time, I still suffered doubts as to whether freedom from fear was actually possible for me. I was absolutely convinced that my case was different. This is a normal reaction when people are asked to try something out of their normal fixed set of beliefs. Yet my conviction grew that, as a spiritual being in physical form, I'm on this planet to learn key lessons. That being the case, to envision life as a moving, constantly changing picture show in the collective mind of the universe was, at the very least, worthy of an experimental effort. In several areas of my life, such as health and business, I had a tendency to abundantly manufacture fearful emotional energy. To be sure, I experienced what I intensely focused on—more fear. For the first time ever, I began to sense that *my inner mental state* was the creative source of my physical reality.

The energy of fear is a bad partner. So is its companion, worry.

Finally, I concluded that for personal growth and transformation, I needed to take full responsibility for my own learning. This meant taking action to resolve specific psycho-emotional issues that were constantly recurring in my life. To achieve my goals, I needed to deconstruct the framework of habitual negative beliefs, thoughts, and emotional energy that I seemed to be carrying in ample supply. I also needed to bring more optimism and joy into my life. It was at about this time that I began listening daily to comedy tapes while driving in my car. I discovered that comedy was a natural mood-altering substance with highly beneficial side effects. Plus, listening to comedy tapes or watching humorous movies is a specific endeavor anyone can partake of if they want to quickly "switch off" the F-E-A-R channel. Try it and I guarantee you'll feel an immediate boost in energy working on your behalf.

A testable experiment in eliminating fear.

In building up my confidence to divert the negative energy of limiting fearful beliefs, once again I "harmonically converged" with Yogananda and his basic concepts. Yoga was something I had been keenly interested in for many years. But could the concepts of this Yogi, who believed in the limitless power of the human mind and the great creative power of inner Spirit, actually work to dismantle fear in the "real" world? Was Yogananda's simple cinematic concept yet another ticket to getting a handle on fear? Could a simple mental belief help win the battle over a life-threatening illness that periodically projected strong pictures of fear on the screen of my mind?

Setting the psychological stage for
stopping fear in its tracks

To test Yogananda's "picture show" hypothesis I began to conduct the following testable mental experiment over a period of thirty days. Whenever I felt the need to emancipate myself from damaging symptoms brought on by fear, I chose to perceive the experience as a giant motion picture show—just as a spectator in the audience would sense it. Taking Yogananda's suggestions to heart, you may, as I did, want to ask yourself the following questions:

- In the drama of life, there often is a main role each of us focuses on. What is the role (e.g., victim, victor) I have created, dwell on, and find myself acting out?

- Do I interpret life through a lens of fear and make fear a major part of my life?

- Life is a reflection of my focused beliefs, thoughts, and feelings. Which fearful beliefs and thoughts are affecting my perceptions and experiences?

- Do I really understand that my fearful beliefs are personal interpretations that rule virtually all aspects of my life?

- Am I mindful that my limiting fearful beliefs can lessen the outcome of medical procedures?

- Do I remind myself I'm a conscious co-creator and can deliberately focus on wants and not on don't wants?

- In daily life circumstances, am I ignoring my inner voice? Do I say "yes" when my heart says "no"?

- Do I recognize I experience in life what I mentally focus energy on?

- ° Do I habitually resist fearful circumstances? If so, do I understand that "what I resist is what I experience" and this is an extension of the principle "what you focus on, you experience?"

To end fear for good, use this technique:

- ° Visualize a beam of light (like a large searchlight) shining down from the sky, illuminating the "picture show" below you strongly desire to change.

- ° Following this, imagine yourself stepping outside the emotional role you've created, off the stage and into the audience with the thought: "This is all merely illusion, a play, sensory data apart from me. It is not what it appears. Its images will soon pass as I distance myself emotionally from the performance."

- ° Envision breaking down any mental barriers you've built that impede the flow of the centering belief that, as a conscious co-creator, you have limitless mental power to alter your negative beliefs and thoughts, and therefore, the drama appearing before you as you wish to see it.

Below are two "live performances" of the technique to end fear right NOW!

Example #1:

A friend informed me that the company he had been with for only a brief period of time called and told him of their serious financial difficulty. Emotionally struggling through a costly divorce at the time, this news became yet another issue contributing to his highly pessimistic outlook. To get clear mentally, he decided the best solution was to detach emotionally and observe the situation from a healthier perspective. He agreed to try stepping outside the life drama in which he found himself. He began focusing on what could go right. Flying in the face of pessimistic thoughts, he talked only about solutions. He told himself that his present experiences were only a temporary "glitch," and nothing more. He reminded himself he was not at the mercy of fearful events that appeared to envelop him—unless he believed he was.

He began talking about (a) how it was possible to meet financial anxieties that adverse circumstances trigger; (b) how to honor and express basic human feelings, rather than repress them; (c) how it was natural to have feelings of apprehension in regard to seeking new employment opportunities; (d) successes he had achieved in the past that underscored his positive self-worth, and (e) the number of companies that had sought to hire him before he signed on with his present job.

As a result of taking a more detached, witnessing role—viewing himself as the director of his life —he pragmatically created an optimistic launching pad to realize his objectives. His newly revised mindset worked wonders to boost his emotional well-being and self-worth. He also agreed he was learning something very important by facing and conquering the presumably overwhelming elements of fear. He was reminded of Nietzsche's insightful message, "What doesn't kill you makes you stronger." He listed his inherent attributes—excellent sales and marketing ability and an innate drive toward action—skills many firms seek out. He agreed that by taking full control of his life—viewing himself as the director of his life drama—he learned specific lessons he was meant to learn in order to grow emotionally, physically and spiritually.

My friend's divorce issues are still an ongoing reality. His employment story, however, took a pleasant turn. He held out until he found a firm that fit his special sales and marketing gifts exactly. More importantly, he now has a working awareness of the conflicting energy of fear and how to overcome it.

Example #2:

One day I arrived home to find my family gathered in the backyard in a highly disturbed mental state. The reason? My son had just discovered that the night before, the largest tree in our back yard had been hit by lightening and had split almost in half. A large portion of the severed trunk was resting on the roof of the house. A tree specialist had been called in to examine the injury, and he informed me in a highly impassioned voice, "Mr. Levinsohn, I was just telling your wife that in a few minutes, the rest of this two-ton tree is sure to come crashing down on the roof of your house."

"Really?" I asked, captured momentarily by his dramatic sense of urgency.

"That's right. Take a look. See how a part of the tree has taken out your TV antennas and gutters?"

"What's it going to cost to cut it down and haul it away?" I asked.

"$4,000," he said, without blinking an eyelash.

"What?" I replied, shocked beyond belief.

"Listen," he said in a highly exaggerated tone of voice, "I gotta tell ya, I'm scared half to death even thinking about climbing your tree, let alone having to sit up there and cut it down. Know why?"

"Why is that?" I answered.

"I'll tell ya why," he blurted out. "If I'm gonna put my life on the line, for sure it's worth a helluva lot more than $4,000. I'm risking my life for you mister and I have to tell ya, it's worth a lot more than four grand." Looking back on the event, it seems to me that this fellow's performance was worthy of an Academy Award. He had terrified me and my entire family, and instilled us with a sense of utter powerlessness by his empassioned "act."

Taking a few deep breaths to relax my body and mind, I imagined myself detaching from the motion picture show being played out on the stage in front of me. I also envisioned a white healing light entering the back of my head to relax my entire body from head to foot. Having prepared myself in this manner, I said, "Look, I'm sorry, but I don't make decisions when my emotions are running wild. Plus, $4,000 is an awful lot of money." To center my mind further, I took a few more deep breaths, and with each one I imagined myself breathing out stress and breathing in the energy of relaxation. I also closed my eyes part way and thought to myself several times, "I feel calm and quiet."

Next, I saw myself as the director of this little drama being played out in my back yard. How long did it take me to get to playing the director role? My guess is no more than sixty seconds. I felt like Clark Kent when he steps into a phone booth, changes his clothes, and a few seconds later appears as Superman. At this moment, a voice inside me told me to walk clear around the tree. The first thing that caught my eye was that the back "out-of-view" portion of the tree had hardly been affected at all. The split in the tree appeared greater from the front where the others were viewing it. I reasoned that this guy had to be a real con man. Why do I say that? Because as he was going through his act, he was circling the tree. This meant he saw exactly what I saw.

"Hold on," I thought, "this tree was hit by lightening the night before, and here it is fifteen hours later and it's still standing. And he's telling me that in a few minutes it's going to come crashing down on the house. Hmm."

Returning to the others, I said, "Listen, my immediate plan is to get two more bids. That's it." Then peering directly at the "expert" I said, "I'll let you know if yours is the lowest bid." Mumbling something sinister under his breath—his performance was over—he walked off in a huff.

Two hours later, we had an honest tree specialist look at the damage. His fee was a fraction of the first man's bid. The first thing he did was secure the fallen portion of the tree to two stronger trees with a rope. Then to my surprise he said, "I'll stop by tomorrow to cut it down."

"Any risk it'll fall on the house?" I asked.

"It'll be fine," he said.

One of the most frequent questions I'm asked by those who have been diagnosed with a life-threatening illness is this: "How do I deal with sudden, unanticipated, and highly stressful events—medical or otherwise?" The first thing to understand is this:

You can't show fear or anxiety if the muscles in your body are relaxed and your breathing is slow and smooth.

It's not physiologically possible to be in a fearful frame of mind while you are breathing slowly, smoothly, and deeply, and your body is in a state of relaxation.

Remind yourself that, in a greater sense, you are a spiritual being and immortal. Hence, there is nothing to fear. Still, anchoring self-suggestion in your subconscious mind demands repetition and regular reinforcement. In this way, when you meet a distressing event, you'll be armed to meet it in a calm and composed manner. The potent and lasting power of self-suggestion will help to quiet the mind and allow you to overcome or circumvent adversity. In addition, repetition breeds contentment.

Caution: Do not resist fear! Resistance generates further anxiety, which clouds judgment. Merely continue the above exercises and those in Appendix II and trust that you'll be relieved of conditions that frighten you. Remind yourself that you can trust your new thoughts and mental imagery because "what you focus on, you get."

Does your life have purpose?

In his book *Man's Eternal Quest*, Yogananda suggests that life has a distinct purpose. It's to learn how to use the limitless energy at your command to alter the beliefs behind the role you've assigned yourself. He suggests, "If you take every happening as you would if you were seeing someone else playing it in a motion picture, you will not grieve." This life view has been instrumental in shifting my inner perceptions away from the trivialities of life's daily dramas. The result: I am now consciously aware of higher levels of truth than can be found in the energy-depleting arena of fear, blame, anger, and resentment. Yet it is no simple task to distinguish between these domains intuitively when one is emotionally immersed in life's dramas. It requires an act of will to consciously observe, detach and disidentify from deeply entrenched beliefs and view them through a healthier lens. Yogananda writes in *Man's Eternal Quest*, "The best way to dissociate yourself from your difficulty is to be mentally detached, as if you were merely a spectator, while at the same time seeking a remedy."

As a result of Yogananda's eternal wisdom, I am better able to effectively "de-stress" fear, which at times I felt I was taking intravenously. My new line of thinking has now given me the dynamic power to let go of many false beliefs that I had turned my attention to and allowed to control my life. Knowing that my beliefs about life shape my experiences has energized me to take a much closer look at what I believe is imaginable, and therefore possible, in beating a life-threatening illness. This "can-do" belief has extended into my personal relationships and to virtually all aspects of my life. My new mind-clearing approach has provided me with the power to prevent the needless dissipation of enormous quantities of vital healing energy. Above all else,

My "director" state of mind has energized me to hold myself accountable and responsible for the day-to-day direction my life is taking.

Another clear-cut benefit of the "director" approach (think of this strategy as taking control of your life) is that I find myself "hooked" less often in energy-draining circumstances. In such instances, consciously shifting my perception out of normal sensory data works amazingly well to conserve my energy.

Here is a real-life example:

My cat-scan appointment was scheduled for 2 p.m. It was after 4 p.m. when I was finally admitted. Emotionally, I pictured and expected a worst-case scenario. As I lay down on the exam table, the nurse tried four times to inject the cat-scan dye. I was becoming fearful, disgruntled, and seriously uncomfortable. Finally the nurse found a vein and injected the dye.

The nurse told me to remain in a fixed body position and not to move. I had no idea what was going to happen next. I felt a bit claustrophobic as the machine surrounded me. I was anxious to get the procedure completed. The nurse said it would be about ten minutes more until the doctor could read the results. Hurriedly she left the room. About thirty minutes later, she returned and stated rather dispassionately, "Listen, your lungs show a trouble spot. The doctor needs to look at the area in more detail. I'll have to repeat the entire procedure." Upon completion, I again was asked to wait ten minutes and remain totally immobile. About forty minutes later, the nurse returned. "Is everything okay?" I asked anxiously. Without preamble, she said, "You'll have to wait until you have a chance to talk to your doctor."

"This is the beginning of the end," I thought, catastrophically. *"This is a disaster waiting to happen. I've had a pain in my upper chest region for the last few days. I'll bet that's it. My cousin was diagnosed in exactly the same way. A few months later he was gone."* I wondered, *"Am I next?"*

"Wait a second," I reminded myself. *"I've pigeonholed myself into a belief that's terribly toxic. And that's the world I'm going to attract and experience. Don't even go there,"* I said to myself. *"I'm choosing to live, not to die."*

"Let's face it," I thought, *"To change my 'awfullizing', I need to stop focusing on a steady barrage of worst-case scenarios. If I don't, that's precisely what I'll attract into my life and experience. Limited thinking won't solve my present dilemma, or open my mind, body, and spirit to the possibility of wellness. The agonizing feelings I'm experiencing right now are reflecting the inner belief that I'm powerless to change my medical condition."*

I could feel my thoughts of fear transfer into almost every muscle of my body. *"Yogananda was right,"* I told myself. *"The best way to dissociate yourself from your difficulty is to mentally detach, as if you were simply a spectator, while at the same time seeking a remedy."*

Witnessing the mental framework I was in, I said to myself, *"I have to put an end to my fearful feelings, uptight muscles and shallow breathing. In this life drama playing out, I have to take a victor not a victim role. That's what being a director is all about. After all, if it's true that I'm a deliberate creator, I can automatically attract thoughts and feelings that are constructive, not self-destructive. Most important is, I already contain the seeds of my own healing within me."*

With that sobering self-talk, I decided to practice a simple yoga relaxation technique I had learned many years ago. For the next three to four minutes, I inhaled and exhaled slowly through my nose. Each time as I exhaled slowly, I felt negative stress leaving my body. As I inhaled slowly, I felt revitalizing energy entering my body. As my personal system of beliefs changed, amazingly, my previous stressful and fearful symptoms diminished.

As I slowly inhaled and exhaled, I added the revitalizing sound of *Ommmmmmm* to this exercise. I began to feel my breath moving effortlessly inward and outward like the long slow motion of gentle waves. I started to feel the muscles of my body relax and fear taper off, like clouds passing by.

"Okay, what else can I do?" I asked myself. "Well, I better take a hard look at the helpless and hopeless self-talk I've been habitually sending to myself. I need to confront head-on, my toxic self-talk. I need to remind myself my body responds as I believe it will." I was thinking, "Abraham Maslow was right when he said, 'If the only tool you have is a hammer, you tend to see every problem as a nail.'" In other words, if past ways of thinking are not working, I need to use new, creative mental tools to solve the problem.

At that point, the one thought, a cliché really, that dramatically triggered me to come to grips with my toxic thoughts was: "If you always do what you've always done, you'll always get what you always got." That was a big answer to a demanding situation.

As an added exercise to deal with fear, HeartMath, a California Institute has proven that psychological, emotional and physical wellness begins with love, and that love can lower stress and anxiety. According to HeartMath, reducing fear begins with accentuating positive thinking from your heart. The basis for their anti-stress technique is understanding that love is letting go of fear, thus achieving peace of mind. It seems the Institute has tested and proven that when you feel the energy of love, you actually feel it in your heart, which they believe is the seat of love.

It seems that briefly re-experiencing a loving or nourishing memory as a mental image creates synchronization in your heart-beat in a few seconds. Once this effect has been established, you will find that it lowers stress and anxiety, elevates immune system functioning, lowers harmful stress hormones, lowers blood pressure, and allows you to focus your thoughts better. Studies by HeartMath have demonstrated that over time, anger, resentment, and fear can produce destructive physical effects. On the other hand, emotions such as love and compassion generate "coherent" heart rhythms which sustain health.

Make unconditional love your guiding principle!

So how do you go about having a change of heart rhythm? The idea is to shift your thought-focus to positive feelings such as love, empathy, and caring. The result: your heart rhythms will change almost instantly.

Here is a simple two-minute anti-stress strategy you can practice three times a day to effectively change your heart rhythms in no time at all. Visualize you are breathing in relaxation and breathing out stress. At the same time, imagine a wonderful memory of a loved one, or a bona fide appreciation of someone or something. That's it. This simple exercise can be practiced anywhere, anytime, such as when you are tied up in traffic, at a physician's office, at work, paying your bills, and so on.

Fear is precipitated by your personal interpretation of a stressful event, which forms a matching future experience. Joined with the De-Stressing Technique in Appendix II, this is an extremely powerful approach to have in your back-to-wellness arsenal. Other methods for changing the reality of stressful situations include listening to comedy tapes, listening to music (high frequency sound, i.e. Mozart, Bach), gardening, walking, et al.

The challenge is to identify those beliefs that are attracting fear and anxiety into your life and replace them with those that give you what you strongly desire. Keep in mind that your expectations of a stressful event mandate your response to it. Plainly, whatever you experience, your expectations make it happen. It makes sense, therefore, to begin picturing yourself as evolving with each new challenge you conquer. Tell yourself, "I can reconstruct this life challenge anyway I choose, because I'm a co-creator, a co-partner in physical form, with Universal or God Consciousness. I've created a fearful situation and it's only me who can change it to what I want to experience, starting right here and right now in this present moment." Remind yourself often: "I 'get' what I focus on and what I expect! Inexhaustible energy flows where attention goes!"

The magic power of "belief-detachment" to tackle life's challenges.

The practice of detaching, stepping outside and witnessing an uncomfortable life drama may make it appear that you are simply hiding from the world. Yet you will no longer find yourself at the mercy of emotional energy that binds you to the past—a powerless state of mind. The lesson? Maintaining a high degree of control over your beliefs will relieve you of much of fear's suffering.

In changing your internal focus by bringing the limitless power of your subconscious into play, you'll now picture yourself as an onlooker; a voyeur who merely witnesses an unpleasant performance without being unsettled by it, as you might have been in the past. This new state of mind will relieve you of the burden of expending even one iota of mental energy more than is absolutely necessary in fearful circumstances. Henceforth, you'll view such "incidents" as products of your own highly charged emotional energy—which now YOU direct.

You are the director of your own life drama.

Let's consider, once more, the advantage of assuming the director's role in your daily life. It gives you the freedom to alter the tone of your experience in much the same way that a pianist purposely shifts from playing a frenzied musical piece to a soulful classical composition, whenever a particular biochemical mood hits. The shift in rhythm, tone, and mood, and the resulting change in internal milieu, is due solely to the willful and decisive action of the musician.

Putting yourself in the director's role is the key to the kingdom of self-empowerment. Since you, as a conscious co-creator, bring your thoughts and beliefs alive, and energy flows where attention (focus) goes, when you act as if YOU are the director in your life it releases you to witness the many sides of your fearful reactions rather than merely succumbing to them. Through this practice, I have achieved a higher level of clarity regarding what's truly mportant in life. From time to time, I can actually feel a portion of my Self moving out beyond my limiting beliefs into higher levels of awareness. As a result, I've learned that I'm not stuck in one sequence of events unless I choose to be. My new mental state has made it possible for me to get in touch with and confront the underlying motives behind my harmful fears.

Theodore Roosevelt offered this advice, "I have often been afraid," he said, "but I wouldn't give in to it. I made myself act as if I was not afraid, and gradually my fear disappeared." Notice the operative words, "act as if" in his statement?

P.S.
Ever Wish You Might Have, Always Available, a Real Authority On the Right Thing To Do In All Situations To Turn Your Life and Health Around? Here's the Final Proof of The Pudding:

Chapter 13

Weapons of Mass Construction: Practical Actions to Turn Your Life and Health Around!

"For any speculation which does not at first glance look crazy, there is no hope."

— Physicist Freeman Dyson

The old saying by Shakespeare, "There is nothing good or bad but thinking makes it so," certainly applies to a former attendee of my Quiet Miracles Back-to-Wellness Workshops. A young woman in her early twenties, she was given less than six months to live. During the course of the first workshop session, I asked,

"Tell me something. What've you been focusing your attention on lately?"

"I've been planning my funeral—in vivid detail," she said in a muted, cowering voice.

"Is that so? Well, I have a better idea for you," I replied.

"And, what's that?"

"Well, before I tell you, would you mind telling me a place you've always wanted to travel to?"

"That's easy. I've always wanted to take a trip to Hawaii."

"Okay," I said, "Then how about over the next three weeks of workshop sessions, you change your focus—and start planning a trip to Hawaii—in vivid detail."

"I'll do it!" she said, somewhat surprised, but at the same time thrilled by the suggestion.

Now fast forward about three years.

Bumping into the young lady at the grocery store, I immediately asked if she had taken her dream trip to Hawaii.

"Yep, and it was everything I thought it would be—and a lot more."

"You know," I said, "I'm wondering what exactly you learned from planning and taking that trip."

"I learned to take responsibility for separating myself from my belief and feeling that I was about to die, which in my mind was a foregone conclusion. Mentally, I was going in the wrong direction. I don't have to tell you that living on the brink of disaster is really scary."

"As a cancer defeater myself, I understand." I said. "Care to share with me anything else you learned?"

Clutching my arm, she said, "The bottom line is that instead of focusing all my attention on dying, I began focusing on living—acting as if what I *wanted* was a foregone conclusion. Know what? I got exactly what I focused on! The mind-opening effects of that experience changed my thinking about a whole lot of things. I learned the hard way that I can choose what I want to think and feel—and as a result, what I experience. Over and over, I kept saying to myself, 'Why would I ever want to create beliefs and feelings that attract and create stress and misfortune?'"

"That's impressive thinking. Tell me, do you have any new intentions you're working on?"

"My intention now is to grow old gracefully, which is a true sign that my thoughts and 'The Times They are A-Changin,' as Bob Dylan wrote."

"Good, and as long you hold firmly to the belief and feeling you'll 'grow old gracefully' in all of its exciting details, that's likely what you'll experience. No question, you've learned well how to apply life's most powerful lessons."

After reading this powerful narrative, are you still skeptical that intensely sustained, constructive thoughts and feelings can overcome a seemingly very grim situation? If so, then you might want to ponder this highly instructive and often-repeated message:

Quantum physics is suggesting that nothing is real(ity) until it is perceived as "real(ity)" by an observer.

Each of us lives our lives first in thought. This means that a job, relationship, or financial crisis we involve ourselves in, is internally created, temporary, and alterable. As far as personal health is concerned, until you focus on wellness, it's not likely that it will suddenly materialize in your life. Perception is the true creator that moves events from mere possibility within to something "real" without. "What is now proved," said William Blake, "was once only imagined."

Be honest. Do you ever make it a point to pay close attention to the toxic thoughts you're focusing on? If quantum physics is to be believed, your thoughts create the circumstances you experience in life. They are meant to give you an immediate response system demonstrating that input equals output, i.e., gloom or gladness in, gloom or gladness out.

Perhaps you've lulled yourself into believing you have no range of choices open to turn around unhappy areas in your life. Greg Hicks and Rick Foster, in their book, *How We Choose to be Happy*, state that the number one characteristic of happy people is an earnest focus on being happy. It seems happiness is a skill that can be acquired, not a chance experience.

A thought is a terrible thing to waste.

As another case in point, Gregg Bradden, author of *The Divine Matrix*, (a book which I highly recommend) tells a true story which brings into focus the idea of emotionally visualizing what you desire as an already fulfilled event. It seems a young man with a wife and two small children was failing with what was diagnosed as a fatal disease. Neville, the single-named author of *The Power of Awareness*, suggested the man alter his downcast belief and focus on acting "as if his healing had already taken place." Bradden quotes William Blake's poetry as a model to emulate:

> *All that you behold, tho' it appears Without, it is Within,*
> *In your Imagination, of which*
> *The World of Mortality is but a Shadow.*

With that perennial wisdom in mind, Neville suggested the following to the dying man: "I suggested that in his imagination, he see the doctor's face expressing incredulous amazement in finding him recovered, contrary to all reason, from the last stages of an incurable disease; that he see him double-checking his examination and hear him saying over and over, 'It's a miracle—it's a miracle.'" The outcome: The power of his new, deeply held belief took the dying young man "through the barrier from the unreal to the real." As the ancient saying goes, "If you put fire in your desire, you'll find the finest things out there, first in here!"

Can you see now why it's so critical to mind your daily thoughts and feelings? Don't even think about identifying with your physical symptoms by thinking or saying, "I have (cancer, heart disease, hypertension, smoking issues, etc). If such verbal venom is a constant presence in your life, remind yourself, "I am what I think and feel. What I focus energy on, I get."

You're probably wondering, "Okay, so what happens if all of my senses are 'telling' me that a particular set of serious circumstances simply can't be changed. Then what?" Answer: With conscious intent, convince yourself that even though your sensory organs may tell you that a physical condition is unalterable, know that, as a conscious co-creator, you have the energy and power within to alter the toxic belief and feeling behind the condition. What you can cause, you can un-cause. After all, you're an aspect of your soul (Universal Consciousness) and you are here to learn how to use your power as a conscious co-creator. This is something you were meant to do naturally and become highly proficient at. Be mindful that the interior challenges you face are always spiritually beneficial. They lead you toward greater personal growth and development.

Only YOU...

Only YOU can make a difference in your life. Only YOU can transform YOU into a self-determining individual. Only YOU can stand up as an advocate for yourself as needed. Only YOU can uncover the toxic beliefs going on in your mind. Only YOU can jumpstart your life. Only YOU can do what others believe is "unthinkable." Only YOU can live your life with fierce determination, refusing to be a victim. Only YOU can live with an air of self-empowerment.

Right about now, you may be thinking you're being sold a bill of "false hope." Would you care to hear physician and author Bernie Segal's response when he was accused of just that by a fellow physician? "There is no such thing as false hope," he said, "there is only false no hope."

Looking to bring your life to life?
Maybe your thoughts and feelings are
holding you hostage!

What the conscious mind asks for, it experiences, so don't be afraid to probe your system of beliefs in search of attitudes that may be undermining your health or inhibiting your recovery. Keep reminding yourself, "I have as my heritage, a divine oneness with Ultimate Consciousness, the Ground of All Being. I am individualized consciousness with unlimited resources. I have the ability to tap into the core of my vast psyche to create the events I want to experience." As you become more and more efficient at this, you'll become ever more grateful for the Divine Presence that you have within you. The Greeks recognized this presence, which is why the Shrine of the Oracle at Delphi was engraved with the simple advice,

"Know Your Self"

Ever wonder what your part in life's great adventure was meant to be? Only you can answer that question, but Andy Andrews, author of *The Traveler's Gift*, points out, "The only limit to your realization of tomorrow is the doubt to which you hold fast today."

The French philosopher Voltaire said, "No snowflake in an avalanche ever feels responsible." Once you become more fully aware of the powers you have within you, you may want to be one of the few snowflakes primed to take responsibility for changing the path of a destructive avalanche heading your way. As Shakti Gawain says in her book, *Creative Visualization*, "The most powerful thing you can do to change the world is to change your own beliefs about the nature of life, people, reality, to something more positive…and begin to act accordingly."

So what's the transformational secret required to max out positive change in your life? It boils down to using your power as a conscious co-creator to discipline yourself to visualize with strong emotion the reality you want to form. The Back-to-Wellness strategies detailed in Appendix II are designed to teach you how. And "The Reality Formation Equation" below will get you started, and make it crystal clear that The Center of Power is YOU.

The Reality Formation Equation:
Visualize. Feel. Act As If. Allow. Dream.

Devote just five minutes, twice a day, with an action-based mindset, to the following simple tasks:

   (a) **Visualize** mentally, in lavish detail, the experiences you want to enter your life.

   (b) **Feel** what you are imaging in your mind firmly as an already completed event. (Remember: The intensity of these thoughts will determine how rapidly they become real.)

   (c) **Act** as if what you desire is already a reality in your life. Plain and simple: "Fake it until you make it!"

   (d) **Allow,** do not resist positive change.

   (e) **Dream.** Just before you fall off to sleep, describe in detail a difficult matter you would like to have cleared away in your dream state. Keep the matter in mind as you drift off to sleep. Do this every night with strong desire and the incubation dream state will provide the means to solve the challenge.

Let's take a few moments and examine how damaging, self-suggestive thoughts and feelings can inhibit physical and spiritual growth by inevitably bringing its own punishment. The following example is based on actual *Quiet Miracles* workshop events. Only the name of Lydia has been changed.

Lydia, a tall, middle-aged woman, decided to attend one of my *Quiet Miracles* workshops. She had just gone through a contentious divorce. Seven days later, she was fired from her job. With these seemingly unsolvable problems facing her each day, Lydia developed an impressive list of dire and all-consuming beliefs: (1) "I'll never get over my personal and financial problems, ever." (2) "I'm sure I'll never get hired again." (3) "There's no possibility that without a job, I can afford to give my two teenage daughters what they deserve, since my former spouse rarely sends money, even though the court says he's supposed to." (4) "For sure, no one will ever fall in love with me." (5) "There's nothing I can do to change the misery in my life." (6) "I'm a failure as a wife and mother." (7) "I'm entirely too thin-skinned and easily hurt." (8) "I'm terribly lonely. I have no one to talk to who really understands my situation." (9) "It's almost impossible to find new friends."

Read Carefully How These Nine Life Choices Will Completely Shape Lydia's Life!

This collection of intensely catastrophic thoughts was likely to be not only self-defeating, but also self-fulfilling. Lydia was clearly selling herself short. Sort of makes you reassess the ancient adage, "It is done unto you as you believe."

If Lydia had chosen to stand apart from and monitor her harmful beliefs instead of dwelling on them, she would have noticed what limited options for growth she was presenting to herself. But because she was giving primary focus to the "evidence right in front of my eyes" (as Lydia described her life), her sensory organs were confirming her strong, hopeless beliefs as "facts of life"—though you can see by re-reading the list, they were merely projections and gloomy predictions rather than in any way *real*.

Yet this did not stop Lydia's stomach from churning when meeting friends and family. She began to believe that others saw her as an abject loser, and fearful her reputation would suffer, she became even more withdrawn. Her friends and family began to wonder if she would ever escape the toxic emotional environment she had created for herself and turn her life around.

To add further force to Lydia's toxic beliefs, she had almost daily fights with her ex-husband over spousal support, children's visitation rights, late payments, why he had abruptly walked out on her, and so on.

Lydia's tendency to expect misfortune to strike at any time showed itself one day when she was advised in a workshop session to try listening to comedy tapes as a means of brightening her spirits. She immediately quoted a joke by comic Steven Wright, known for his dead-pan delivery. Meeting a beautiful woman in a bar, Wright was asked, "How do you feel?" His answer, "Well, you know when you're sitting on a chair and you lean back so you're just on two legs, then you lean too far and you almost fall over, but at the last second you catch yourself? I feel like that all the time."

With dark thinking and dead-pan delivery, Lydia removed the possibility of joy entering her life almost entirely. She chose not to accept the idea that it might be worthwhile to examine her beliefs, in the hope of identifying, and changing, the patterns of thought that were shaping her life.

According to strict definition, Lydia was dysfunctional. To further compound matters, one year after her divorce, Lydia was diagnosed with cancer. At this point her response was to renounce life altogether, wall herself off in her small apartment, and nurse the conviction that she was helpless and unable to cope with life. By conscious choice, she rendered herself powerless. What she failed to "see" was this omnipresent Law of Nature: *The universe is always conspiring to give you what you believe, think, expect and feel.*

Fortunately, Lydia was persuaded in no uncertain terms by her daughters and friends to take corrective action to turn her life around, and quickly! What she had yet to learn was the wisdom of John Wooden who said, "Failure to act is often the biggest failure of all."

Repairing the damage.

Overwhelmed, not knowing what to expect from a workshop "full of strangers," Lydia had almost to be dragged physically by her two teenaged daughters to her first *Quiet Miracles*, Back-to-Wellness session. In spite of the nurturing support of workshop attendees, Lydia could see no good reason for her presence there. Looking and behaving much like a victim, she did a masterly job of bringing down the energy level of the entire group by drawing other attendees into her world of unnerving negative assumptions.

At first this behavior served as a harsh object lesson for workshop attendees concerning the harm of identifying with your damaging beliefs and feelings. It immediately became evident that Lydia was unwilling to explore the principles of the workshop. Yet, because other attendees had begun to develop strong belief in their own self-value, they extended that belief to

Lydia. In time, Lydia began to hear her destructive self-talk with new ears. She also began to understand what a destructive message such thoughts and emotions were sending to the cells of her body—and the universe at large.

Lydia had legitimate questions she wanted answered. "C'mon now," she declared, "you can't be serious when you tell me that most anything is possible in life. Look, I simply don't believe science is saying that nothing happens until I personally 'see' it as a possibility—as actually happening."

"That perception is limiting your world," would be the reply. "You need to move outside that dis-belief. Given enough intensity your thoughts come true."

"Yeah, well one thing I know for sure," countered Lydia, "Taking any kind of control over my life has been totally beyond me. I've tried. It's never worked."

An astute workshop attendee piped in and said, "Maybe you need to pay attention to how you're feeling and understand that emotions create your life experiences and that whatever you think and feel comes right back at you."

Regular doses of peer pressure from attendees who had "been there, done that," prompted Lydia, at some soul level, to begin to understand that her emotions follow her thoughts, beliefs and expectations. Pushed gently forward by workshop attendees, but often hesitant to take a hard look at her destructive core beliefs and change them, she finally chose to take off the shutters and peer closely at her defective, non-working and contradictory beliefs. With a burst of evocative revelation, Lydia awakened to the idea she was not helpless, nor was she inferior, but was given the gift of conscious co-creation for a reason: To generate dynamic energy to manifest the life events she most wanted to experience. Owing to the never-ending inspiration and all-embracing concern of other attendees, Lydia acknowledged that her belief in helplessness was being physically reflected back to her in the stark form of uncomfortably dark life experiences.

Workshop rules (beliefs) to live by:
No dumping allowed!

To prevent a deeply depressed workshop member's toxic expectations from affecting the energy of others, several attendees suggested that basic back-to-wellness rules ought to apply to each workshop session in order to prevent energy deflators from taking over. Attendees "spare-me-your-negative-drama" rules included (a) Using a 5 minute timer to limit the time anyone can talk about their troubles. (b) Not using other workshop members as a crutch, since each attendee has available to him or her, the natural power of conscious co-creation. (c) A $1.00 charge for whining, negative body language, depressed tone of voice, faraway facial expressions, overly-gloomy outlook, one-upmanship, put-downs, failing to admit wellness is a possibility, or meddling, unless asked. It was decided that monies collected be donated to a worthwhile cause. The above "rules" helped attendees with a downer persona make each day appear new again by creating a controlled therapeutic workshop environment—which attendees were reminded to start creating at the start of each day on their own.

Extreme makeover: Long story short!

Lydia could hardy help noticing that being part of a can-do workshop group is not only an ongoing, life-altering resource, but a way to venture out and meet interesting and empathetic people willing to invest in her fate. Digging a little deeper and listening to insightful workshop feedback, Lydia admitted she was the prime author of her past sorrows. She was appropriately reminded of the old saying, "If it's in the way, it is the way." To take conscious creation a step further, it was suggested that Lydia look around at the negative events in her life and understand they were not forced upon her; they were focused on by her, they were formed by her, and she needed to take personal responsibility for originating them.

When hesitating to make changes in her self-destructive mindset, Lydia was reminded repeatedly, "If not now, when?" which she saw powerfully demonstrated by other attendees. She noticed too that their existential "No Excuses" system of beliefs created victors and not victims, which she found highly contagious.

Summoning her courage at long last, Lydia accepted the legitimacy of her feelings as feelings and agreed not to bottle them, but to track them daily with the knowledge they represent her own subjective feelings about reality and not inevitable reality itself. More than once she heard, "Yes, Lydia, the emotions you feel are real! They exist as a natural outcome of your system of beliefs. They surface as matching life events and are of your own making."

It was suggested to Lydia that she challenge her damaging core assumptions by putting the Back-to-Wellness Techniques (see Appendix II) to the test; to actually use them for 30 days. She welcomed the challenge. Lydia now accepts as "fact" that when she alters her belief in powerlessness, the physical "proof" confirms her new belief as dramatically as it did her toxic one. She says that a true transformative experience occurred when she realized she herself created the perspective that she was a victim of circumstances she had created.

Lydia now sensibly realizes that when she alters a thought in the present moment, she simultaneously changes the past and probable future. She is learning to believe in the vast creative power of every ongoing thought. A big AHA for Lydia is recognizing that if the past, present, and future are taking place simultaneously, which the new science is suggesting, then rooting herself firmly in past thoughts and feelings of depression in the present only seeds the future with more of the same, all of which can be hazardous to her health and well-being. With new and healthy beliefs, a new commitment to life, a deepening spiritual faith, a will to live, and a new sense of purpose, along with expressions of love to family and friends, Lydia says she is proud of the courage and responsibility she is displaying each day in dealing with her personal challenges.

Today, Lydia, having established a new relationship with herself, understands that fearful events that enter her life are the end result of her depressing and damaging thoughts and expectations. She recognizes that when she feels a sense of helplessness and hopelessness, she is open to tell herself, "I feel helpless," while acknowledging also that this feeling is not a "fact of life", but a sensation generated by her destructive thoughts, which need to be revamped. It would be folly to act as if such feelings do not exist. Worse than that, it would make it impossible for her to uncover the destructive beliefs causing them. Lydia is then to ask herself, "Why do I feel a sense of helplessness and hopelessness?"

Improving each day in small increments, Lydia is learning that the present moment is her most active point of creative power; that the present is where all creation occurs. And, as a human and divine co-creator, she has power in each present moment to alter the past and all probable future events, all of which are open to change.

Lydia is advised to awaken each morning with an air of excitement, "knowing" she possesses the gift of conscious co-creation and hence, the ability to take control of her life. It's suggested that she list, item by item, events she wants to bring into her life and to then imagine and feel each of them as a *fait accom-pli*, a thing already done, a "done deal."

Constructing a "Done-Deal" List!

Feeling in greater control of her destiny, Lydia decided to create a file on her computer, listing item by item each experience she wanted to enter her life as an accomplished event. She made a private contract with herself that, "Every day, I will focus intently on each item on my list, vividly envisioning and feeling what it's actually like to experience it in my life as an already "done deal". Each morning upon awakening Lydia starts afresh, strengthening her beliefs with clearly-defined circumstances she dramatically wants to experience. She understands she will succeed in direct proportion to the mental effort she expends. Twice each day she focuses intensely on each item on her "Done-Deal" list of high expectations, telling herself with childlike vision, "Letting go of the old, I now believe and actually feel the positive outcome of each item I want to create as a 'done deal,' a 'fact' of life! So be it!"

Caution:

Don't let a twice daily "Done Deal" opportunity slip by. Keep in mind that one strong expectation will register as a completed event to an extent far greater than many mere wishes or desires. Confine yourself to generating thoughts and feelings that enrich your soul and that evidence your power as a conscious co-creator. Your "Done-Deal" List will be your daily sanctuary—a safe port out of the storm—because with each practice session, you'll become more finely attuned to the deep, inner guidance of Universal or God Consciousness.

Finally, Lydia was advised at the workshops to look for opportunities to get involved in helping others, as one further means of changing her focus, and she has recently begun doing volunteer work with cancer patients.

At this point in her journey, Lydia is becoming increasingly confident that,

**The exterior of your life expresses the
condition of the interior.
YOU form the reality you know!
YOU consciously choose what you want to focus on
and, as a natural consequence, what you experience.**

To liberate life's highest possibilities, James Allen stated the following basic law of nature: "You are today where your thoughts have brought you; you will be tomorrow where your thoughts take you." That's the glory of knowing you possess creative powers all your own that can carry you over virtually any obstacle. Make no mistake about it. Wishing won't do it. Only taking aggressive action will. Your power as a responsible conscious co-creator is within. To have it working for you to form the life you desire, you need only draw on its powers, which contain all possibilities.

The Soul Agreement
For Your Eyes Only!

"A single gentle rain makes the grass many shades greener. So our prospects brighten on the influx of better thoughts."
             – Henry David Thoreau

Look and you will find it—what is unsought will go undetected."
             – Sophocles

The Soul Agreement

Whereas, quantum physics suggests I am an immortal, creative, spiritual being, and;

Whereas, being a self-critiquing reality checker, I believe firmly that thoughts and feelings are energy-power, and that inner intention is a wellness trail blazer, a key navigator to open doors that I may not presently know exist, and;

Whereas, I have cosmic permission to mold the fluid-like energy around me with every focused thought I think and vividly imagine with strong feelings, and;

Whereas, I am fully cognizant of the tremendous pressure to avoid looking within to eradicate my self-sabotaging, uncensored toxic beliefs, thoughts, expectations and feelings;

Therefore, Be it Resolved that from this day forward, I shall empower myself to rise to this overwhelming challenge to wash away old self-limiting boundaries, and with lion-like courage and determination, set out to establish and achieve my vision-expanding goals of wellness on all levels of my being, emotional, physical and psychological. Moreover, I will apply hidden reserves of fierce intention to the task of living and breathing wellness, through the daily practice of outcome-oriented visualization, the suspension of damaging thoughts technique, prayer-dream therapy, meditation, and like approaches and, through cajoling, sweet-talking and positive self-talk, convince myself that I am a worthy human, an individualized aspect of Divine Consciousness and a conscious co-creator that most assuredly deserves wellness benefits, just as others have who have beaten a serious illness.

Whereas, I recognize that if my thoughts and feelings are healthy, and daily I rehearse success, the world will match what I perceive, since the new science is suggesting that there is no reality until it is perceived reality; and

Whereas, by the same notion, if I project unhealthy beliefs, thoughts, expectations, and feelings, that too is what the world will bestow upon me—for what one resists—persists; and

Whereas, if I perceive life through a lens of anger, unforgiveness, ill health, and the like, the portrait I see will be colored by my font of hair-raising beliefs—which in the sands of time, I will draw to my life by the influences of The Law of Attraction;

Therefore, verily, in this calm-eyed moment, let the epiphanies of toxic thought and feeling dismantling begin! And, armed with strong intention, persistence, and omnipotent ability as a conscious co-creator, let me unleash my energies to savagely attack and renounce any negative outlook and belief-addiction to doom and gloom and with deft mental parries and masterfully skilled ability, day-in and day-out, fiercely pursue and mentally visualize the wellness outcome I intently desire as already achieved, which I now recognize can, through divine mutation, prevent, slow down, stop, and even reverse serious illness.

Whereas, having discerned what long-term survivors achieve via the fertile possibilities of positive imagery and strong feelings, and;

Whereas, the momentum of a strong-willed, optimistic energy field will hold me on a course of wellness and deepest spiritual aspirations;

Therefore, I resolve from this day forward to perform on myself a do-it-yourself toxic belief-overhaul ("Beliefectomy"), and with flailing slashes of self-talk, say "No!" to unforgiveness issues, "No!" to resentment and anger, and "No!" to hopelessness and helplessness and other unregulated inner nemeses that have previously been much out of control. Each day I shall ravenously write 100 times until it is mentally embedded that "I am free of the self-hypnotic hold of past toxic beliefs that have energetically impoverished my psyche and physical body's basic defense mechanism."

Whereas, by order of Divine Intelligence, I am innately designed to celebrate cosmic spiritual development and exploration of life's possibilities on planet Earth—a soul-elevating quest—I recognize that each of us has free will, with all of its rights, powers and emoluments, so that we can, as perceptive beings, make new choices, and that it is our will or intention that chooses and summons forth what subsequently shall come to fruition in our lives; and

Whereas, I recognize that, based on the eternal nature of the soul, life in my physical body is for the venerable purpose of learning higher spiritual lessons of love, compassion and joy; and that by listening to divine intuition, my inner guidance system, I will honor the many gifts I have received;

Therefore, I thereupon resolve to look forward to my ongoing adventures in self-illumination and construct my life exactly as I choose to experience it.

The Quiet Miracles organization and the divine omens, by virtue of these resolutions, and in recognition of the magnitude of signing this binding soul agreement, give this award to individuals who have sounded the clarion call resounding thunderously throughout the universe, that negative beliefs, thoughts, expectations and feelings will, from this time onward, be rendered futile, and do hereby on the signing of this document, proclaim that _____ shall be bestowed

The Edmund Hillary Mount Everest Award

for attainment of climbing to unsurpassed heights in demonstrating to the universe that by taking a mountain top perspective, one can liberate one's imagination of toxic thoughts and feelings, and attain wellness and peace of mind, thus filling oneself with life's full potential, and thereby authenticating the exhilarating ancient counsel that "As you think, so you become."

In Testimony Whereof, I have hereunto set my hand and caused my signature to be affixed in the state of_____ _____ this _____day of _____ the year of our Lord, Two Thousand _____.

_____

Your Higher Consciousness (Soul)

Appendix II

The Modern Fundamentals of Wellness:

12 Powerful Longevity Exercises That
Can Slow Down, Stop, and Even
Reverse Serious Illness

In 1819, Hans Oersted observed that electric currents have magnetic effects. Based on Oersted's discovery, Professor Joseph Henry of Princeton took a piece of iron with no magnetic capabilities and magnetized it by winding insulated wires around its core and charging it with the current from a small battery. The result: The iron became a powerful, highly charged electromagnet that lifted more than 3500 pounds.

You too have at your command a powerful battery with magnetic field strength! And it's thousands of times more powerful than any man-made magnet. What's more, it can multiply your thought and feeling power exponentially to turn your health and life completely around. As you can guess, it's called *The Power of Attraction*. To reclaim your power and put it to use, here are the "Back-to-Wellness" techniques (a literal self-empowerment guide) used by many of the long-term cancer survivors I interviewed.

Lifelong self-empowering tools.

To impact your health and well-being, it's important to keep yourself motivated during the initial period you begin practicing the "Back-to-Wellness" Techniques that follow. For this reason, we have placed emphasis only on basic principles and techniques. This should lighten your load considerably and make getting started much easier. You won't have to be up until the wee hours of the morning searching through the Internet, visiting chat groups and libraries, attending expensive workshops and scratching your head, because long-term cancer survivors have already "been there done that" and discovered what works.

In order to prevent information overload, I've given the daily "Back-to-Wellness" Techniques that follow both an overview and a detailed description. As with anything new, there will be short-term highs and lows. But when all is said and done, I can virtually guarantee you'll learn to leverage your own inner healing to its optimum power, if you invest the time and energy required to put these wellness factors and Techniques to work on a daily basis.

All we ask is that you not be a foot-dragger or a Doubting Thomas, but put yourself on the line (which a chronic illness already has succeeded in doing) and try these proven and time-tested "Back-to-Wellness" Techniques. Others have rekindled the healing process using these Techniques to bring about their own achievement—you can as well.

Reducing to simple English
all the puzzling information "out there."

It's important not to speed-read each essential Wellness Technique. You must take the necessary time to review and practice each on a daily basis. Practice will go a long way to bolstering your confidence and immune response.

Let's clarify one point . . .

The time and intensity you spend on these "Back-to-Wellness" Techniques will dictate your ultimate success. Vince Lombardi, the late, great football coach, once said:

> *The difference between a successful person and others is not a lack of strength, not a lack of knowledge, but rather a lack of will.*

98% of smart is knowing what you're dumb at.

Experience has taught me that if you start with an experimental mindset, you will begin to see new wellness possibilities you never thought existed. You may want to focus on the wisdom of Ralph Waldo Emerson who said, "All life is an experiment. The more experiments you make the better."

The most critically important Wellness Techniques are the Suspension of Damaging Thoughts Technique, the Outcome-Oriented Visualization Technique, and the Prayer/Dream Technique. What about the other techniques detailed? Well, I have certain favorites I resonate with, which I include in my daily regimen and I'm certain you will, too.

What if you already are using your own results-oriented visualization technique or any of the other approaches? No problem. If you incorporate even one or two aspects of the techniques presented here, you'll have at your personal command, life-enriching strategies that work even better for you.

Reminder: Batteries are not included!

Some individuals with chronic illness have the misguided notion that once they've adopted a program, all they have to do is sit back passively and wait for something good to happen. But I have stressed throughout this book that willful intent and intensity will be required to take control of your medical journey. The inner summons must come from you.

Many years ago, Napoleon Hill wrote an essay called "The Habit of Going the Extra Mile." The title really says it all. When you've contracted a chronic illness, this burning drive is even more essential. Personal initiative is a skill that can be learned, and one that's essential to conquering illness.

The twelve essential life-enhancing "Back-to-Wellness" Techniques, followed by a Daily Action Plan, are meant to inspire you to better health and well-being. I've added several survival suggestions that have expanded on the teachings of Claude Bristol, who wrote a wonderful book I highly recommend entitled *The Magic of Believing.*

Making wellness happen requires attention and effort on your part! There is no way around the idea that in all of life, "You get what you focus on!"

Twelve Powerful "Back-to-Wellness" Techniques that Demonstrate How to Chart a New Path to Wellness

Wellness Exercise #1:
The Suspension of Damaging Thoughts Technique

When you're diagnosed with a life-threatening illness, the life challenge is to cultivate the determined attitude of long-term survivors who defy all scientific odds. As part of the wellness process, and to empower you against feelings of helplessness and hopelessness—you first must learn how to uncover the root causes (core beliefs) behind your negative thoughts and feelings, speak to them directly and suspend them (frequently this takes professional assistance, which I strongly encourage you to seek out).

During this exercise, you'll be asked to put aside your deeply rooted beliefs about chronic illness or virtually any crisis. You'll be shown in simple language, actual proof that it's possible to triumph over the beliefs and thoughts that can undermine your health.

First a little background on this technique: Two friends, one a well-known physician and the other a prominent attorney, have long been interested in Eastern philosophy, and both are regular practitioners of yoga meditation. Both friends note that any conscious attempt to suppress harmful thoughts largely strengthens them. For the past thirty years, their practice of meditation has taught them that when you witness your mind holding a thought, it allows that thought to dissipate, much like a bubble rising to the surface of a lake and bursting. In this way the debilitating thought loses its destructive energy and fades out of present reality.

The life lesson here is to *witness* rather than becoming involved with or attached to contaminating thoughts.

"In other words," my physician friend says, "the idea is to observe or witness the damaging thought as an object separate from yourself. Freed of the psycho-emotional energy of dysfunction, your body can open itself to positive energies that heal."

To stop and replace damaging thoughts, practice the following Suspension of Damaging Thoughts Technique three times a day:

1. Examine your damaging thoughts and feelings (messages you send to yourself daily such as feelings of hopelessness and helplessness, unwillingness to forgive someone, anger).

2. Say STOP (envision a STOP sign).

3. Argue with the damaging thought.

4. Change your toxic self-talk, i.e., For the next seven days, focus on what can go right. Then for another seven days, ad infinitum.

5. Replace your toxic thoughts with joyful self-affirmations, for example, "Every day in every way I AM perfectly healthy."

6. Mentally picture on the screen of your mind the results you want to enter your life and are affirming as already achieved.

7. FEEL and act as if the outcome you strongly desire is a present "fact" of life.

Robert Jaffe, a medical doctor mentioned earlier, who has worked with patients with life-threatening illnesses said it best, "Healing isn't about fixing symptoms. It's about discovering its root cause and addressing it directly." As an example, let's look at the before-and-after effect of the following emotionally expressive statement—truly a strong barrier to healing. Notice how the highly potent belief empowers feelings of hopelessness and helplessness:

"Sure, I'd like to get well. That's pretty obvious. But I'm driven to think only about my poor health."

To counter that energy-blocking conflicting belief and reduce its empowering energy to inflict bodily damage, say to yourself,

"I'm going to suspend that thought for now. Instead, I'm going to implant the thought, 'Every day in every way, I am perfectly healthy.'"

The next step is to add a large dose of desire and persistence. Your own internal resources as a conscious co-creator will strengthen and evolve, and take you to the wellness place you're envisioning. Remind yourself that thoughts are vibrating energy. They are real(ity) in time and space.

Thoughts and the feelings they generate convey a form of oscillating energy. The greater the intensity of the belief and thought, the more radiant the physiologic effect on body chemistry. Like drawing energy from an inspirational speech or strong emotional tension, thought-energy can act positively or negatively. Therefore by taking responsibility for and altering your sabotaging beliefs, thoughts, and feelings, you automatically take charge of your healing journey.

Wellness Exercise #2:

The Outcome-Oriented Visualization Technique

"For those who believe, no proof is necessary.
For those who do not believe, no proof is possible."

– Anon

It's my belief that this technique saved my life. I'm convinced it was through "imaging" myself as already healthy and cancer-free three times a day—with intense feeling and undivided focus—that I became well. Cultivating this technique changed my entire mental focus, transforming me into a person who could take control of his attitude and life conditions with strength and power, even in the most unfavorable circumstances. Through regular practice, you'll become familiar with this feeling as well. Practice the visualization exercise for thirty days and you'll discover the ease with which you can achieve a state of almost total relaxation, bringing perfect peace and restful calm.

If you read nothing else about how wellness actually works—read this! It is what everyone ought to know about how to solve challenges you believe are unsolvable.

It's been acknowledged by medical science that white blood cells (WBCs) have neuroreceptors on their surface that respond immediately to beliefs, thoughts, and emotions (feelings are chemicals, remember?). The mental images you focus on communicate instantly, via molecular messengers, with your body's basic defense system. Such messages can block or enhance healing.

Since your WBCs kill cancer cells, viruses, and bacteria, it's clear that your thoughts play an important role in maintaining

226

your health. By taking charge of the picture-forming power of your mind you can maintain healthy immune functioning.

The mental impression I find simplest to imagine is picturing the thymus gland (an organ located in the chest cavity that produces white blood cells) producing large quantities of natural killer (NK) cells. I watch as they move directly into my bloodstream and swim to all parts of my body. Next, I picture my NK cells acting as powerful magnets, drawing to them, and neutralizing all cancer, virus infected or abnormal cells in my body.

Before you get started on this important self-empowering back-to-wellness technique, however, it may be a good idea to get an actual picture of your cat scan or x-ray to give your mind a vivid mental representation of the abnormal cell area(s). In my own case, the doctors made a serious effort to explain the specific whereabouts of any abnormal cells in my body. This gave me an extremely clear mental picture of the areas that required wellness imagery.

Next, find a time and place where, three times a day, you can be alone. One session should take place in the morning, when you're not quite fully awake. At this time, your mind is still in what I call the "hypnogogic sleep zone"—a time when your subconscious is more apt to be open to the power of self-suggestion. In addition, you have not yet entered the day. The hassles and problems of everyday life can more easily be shut out. Another session should take place at night just before going to sleep. This way, your mind continues to work on scenes of wellness 24 hours a day. This can be instrumental in inciting the body's defenses into action. The third session should take place in the afternoon when you're a bit tired and receptive to autosuggestion. Obviously you must work around your own schedule.

To a large degree, learning to visualize wellness is like learning most things—it must be done in gradual steps. Compare the process to learning to play an instrument. You must first practice the scales, over and over, before playing Mozart.

Go at your own pace, but try to inject fun and joy into each session, without losing sight of the need to practice with emotional intensity.

The visualization exercise detailed here is a step-by-step program that can have a major impact on your ability to deal with a life-threatening illness or other crisis in your life. It is meant to supplement, not replace, allopathic medicine. This exercise is broken into several segments:

(1) A constant stream of positive mental images which physiologically foster wellness,

(2) a brief explanation as to why certain key beliefs are included in the exercise, and

(3) important comments to help you restore healthier emotional states by encouraging you to look at best case expectations.

Remember that in all of life, you experience what you focus on and expect. Therefore, to maintain your innate power to elicit greater health and reduced emotional stress, you should practice this technique three times a day. Initially, you may want to tape record the script below and play it back for two or three practice sessions. This will help enhance your images and feelings of wellness, so your awareness energy will surpass the area requiring wellness. When you're comfortable with the process, discard the tape and use your own beliefs and internal imagery to promote wellness.

Though the health-promoting script below may appear somewhat long in print, once you begin marshalling this powerful mind-body communication technique, it can protect your health without your ever being aware of the subtle changes taking place both emotionally and physically. A condensed alternative visualization exercise will also be provided for your consideration.

IMPORTANT: After several sessions, feel free to simply employ the ten to one count-down to place yourself in a relaxed state of mind, then skip directly to the TV screen. You should not lose sight of the main objective: focusing on the beliefs, feelings and mental images essential to restoring your health. An aside: a number of workshop attendees seem to expend far too much energy before arriving at the TV screen.

The whole idea is to aim your powerful beliefs and feelings at intensely visualizing the outcome you want to achieve as completed.

A single visualization session will take, at the very most, no more than five minutes. I timed several sessions and found after approximately one week of practice, I could complete an entire back-to-wellness session in less than four minutes. Less really is more.

Before you begin, set yourself a creative challenge. For thirty days, with positive expectation and strong feeling, earnestly and persistently practice the outcome-oriented visualization exercise three times a day. You'll discover that through your own self-suggestive responsiveness, the limiting beliefs and thoughts you have resigned yourself to will begin to fall away.

And don't be afraid to conjure up the ***best possible*** outcome you can envision as an already completed event.

Let's begin:

Step 1 — Getting Ready

To begin your visualization session sit spine straight, shut your eyes, cup your hands in your lap, and take several deep breaths to relax any body tension (particularly your face and neck muscles). Then, as you inhale through your nose (mouth closed), think belly OUT, chest OUT. As you exhale through your nose (mouth closed), think belly IN, chest IN. As you exhale, feel stress leaving your body. As you inhale, feel revitalizing energy entering your body.

Now, add the sound of Om (OH-mmmm) either silently or in a whisper as you both inhale and exhale, e.g., Ommmmm-mmmm. Don't focus on the sound. Merely be aware of it. If you find your mind wandering or hear external sounds, gently bring your awareness back to the sound of Ommmmmmmmmm. This detached, witnessing principle is essential to achieving optimum results. Try to cease resisting fearful or mind-wandering images. Resisting may only focus more of your thoughts on those images. Don't attempt to relax. Let it happen. You'll notice the more you practice, the easier it gets.

The idea is to feel your breath moving effortlessly inward and outward like the long slow motion of gentle wavelets. During the exercise tell yourself, "My mind, my body and my breath are breathing as one, together in a wonderful state of harmony."

Step 2:

Continue this exercise for eight to ten inhale/exhale cycles until you feel moderately free of mental distractions and mind-wandering. Observe your breath naturally flowing in and out of your nose. This will help shut out the outer world while opening a gateway to invoke Infinite Energy from your inner being. Your internal chanting, along with witnessing the flow of your breath and the interlude between breaths, will tend to subdue wandering thoughts so they become calm, peaceful, and "out of mind."

Step 3:

See yourself walking toward an imaginary Healing Temple, a place you know will restore your health. When you approach, a wide gate opens and you enter. Once inside the gate, the first thing you notice is a moving walkway. You step on the walkway and are magically taken to the front door of the Healing Temple. You step up and ring the bell. The door opens, but you see nothing. A calm voice invites you in and asks you to state your request. You respond by saying, "I would like Spiritual Guidance on ridding myself of _____ (the life challenge you desire to conquer)."

Next, you see a guide—someone who matters a great deal to you. This guide could be a spouse, friend, or parent—someone who is with you now or who has passed on. (For simplicity's sake, I'll refer in the exercise to that person as female, although it doesn't mean your guide must also be female.) The person approaches and hugs you. There is a serenity in this deeply, emotional moment...a sublime kind of elation. She leads you to an Ancient Healing Room. You walk up a short staircase and into the special room. At once, you sense that the room emits an unmistakable calm, working its healing magic to induce ease and relaxation. The Ancient Healing Room is large and inviting, like an oversized living room. Subdued lighting and thick, earth-toned carpet complement the room. Floating in the air, barely perceptible, are soft sounds of nature—wind, tropical surf, and birds—like voices of reassuring serenity. The mahogany walls of the room are lined from floor to ceiling with books on healing by the world's greatest healers from ancient to modern times.

Sitting in the center of the room is a giant TV set with a 75-inch monitor. Directly in front of the TV set is a large, comfortable couch. There's a TV camera on one side. You find a comfortable, upright position on the couch.

Step 4:

Your guide asks you to watch the 75-inch TV monitor in the middle of the room. You notice she selects a channel marked "Present Tense" on her oversized remote control. The TV monitor blinks on and is immediately framed in revitalizing white light. Simultaneously, the TV camera on the side of the couch clicks to on, and all at once you see your thymus gland producing natural killer (NK) cells, which have the capability to kill virus-infected cells and neutralize cancer cells. You see a release of large quantities of NK cells from your thymus gland move directly into your bloodstream. Visualize the cells swimming and binding, like powerful magnets, to all abnormal cells in your brain and body, neutralizing them. As you peer closer, you see all disease-causing cells vanish. Confidently, you see your body in perfect health—and all parts working flawlessly in harmony. A sense of self-empowerment and peace of mind comes over you. You feel good knowing your NK cell defense system is in place and operating around the clock to protect you.

You now see yourself framed in a white healing light, acting with boundless energy, fully restored to health and emotional well-being. You feel yourself enveloped in this white healing light for several minutes.

Next, your guide punches a button on the remote control for a TV channel marked "Future Event." She asks you to watch the monitor where again you picture your health totally restored. You "see" yourself with unlimited vitality and exuberant optimism. You feel that no obstacle can hold you back as you suddenly realize you are part of Infinite Energy Itself.

Once again, your guide asks you to look at the TV monitor surrounded by white healing light. She says, "What you are about to witness now is a visit with your physician after you have completed all of your treatments." (The specifics of this event will depend on the life challenge you are seeking to conquer.) Anxious, you look up at the giant monitor and see your doctor. He's telling you that all abnormal cells are gone. Eliminated. You see yourself thanking the doctor, clenching your fist and saying "Yes!" in a kind of emotionally intense "high five" or "Hallelujah!" gesture.

Then your guide clicks off the TV monitor and asks, "What life lessons are you learning from this experience?" You think about this and respond honestly. Perhaps you have learned that during the most troubling times, we have the greatest opportunity for personal growth. Perhaps it's that you should better focus your life and try to accomplish things—large and small—that are far more meaningful, noble and worthwhile, and that would help others.

Your guide then asks, "Do you have any new goals?" Again, you answer honestly. Perhaps your goal is to bring the powerful force of love into your inner being by forgiving someone, exhibiting less anger, helping others, or becoming a better father, mother, daughter, son, grandparent, friend, or citizen. Your guide is proud and tells you that the healing session is now over. She walks with you through the Ancient Healing Room to the exit door of the Temple. Outside, you both step onto the moving sidewalk that takes you to the outer gate. You hug goodbye.

Automatically, the wide gate closes behind you. Standing outside the gate, you say to yourself, "Every day in every way, I AM perfectly healthy." Slowly, you count from one to ten suggesting to yourself you'll awaken refreshed and re-vitalized. You open your eyes. The visualization session is over.

Incidentally, you can obtain a picture of the thymus gland from any library. It is an organ located in the chest cavity that produces white blood cells for the immune response. Take a mental picture of the thymus before you begin the exercise so the mental impressions you produce are clear in your mind. This is the internal image you want to see on the TV monitor of your mind.

**It's extremely important to practice
the entire visualization exercise three times a day.**

Caution: Practicing extra sessions demonstrates you have doubts the outcome-oriented visualization technique will work. With confidence and expectation, effortlessly experience each three-a-day session, acting as if what you're envisioning is an already completed event. And then put the session out of your mind. To begin to change your exterior well-being, it's essential to focus your mind on new, healthy beliefs and thoughts. Constructive thoughts, repeated often enough, increase your likelihood of attracting what you focus attention on. Refrain from worrying about bills that need to be paid, the laundry, the kids, the mortgage. Any time such thoughts enter your mind, be patient with yourself. Reassure yourself that this is your time for healing, and that you'll think about such matters later. Trust your new beliefs, and shortly, your mind will "click" into your back-to-wellness mental images, and with repeated practice, sustain them. Be persistent. Keep practicing. Expect you'll succeed and, through your new vision, the body's physiological processes will convert your images into a matching likeness.

What do you believe is the key element in the visualization exercise?

The most important component of the visualization exercise is intensely picturing your immune system's natural killer cells neutralizing cancer cells, virus-infected cells, or abnormal cells. Visualize your body's NK cells pouring out of the thymus gland into your bloodstream. See them swimming and binding to all abnormal cells in your brain and body.

Mental pictures conveyed with heightened emotional intensity bring the mental impressions you envision to life.

The depth of feeling behind the mental impressions you create is the essential element to inciting the subconscious mind to actualize your mental imagery. Emotional intensity is the ammunition required to fuel realization of your mental pictures of wellness. What I've discovered is the greater the emotional desire of my mental imagery, via positive mental images and heightened expectation, the shorter the incubation period to realization. Confidently seeing your body in perfect health and harmony is also critical to actualizing your new beliefs.

Your physical body is chemically altered with your every thought!

Each cell in your body is listening to your every thought and reacting accordingly. Be mindful that either you rule your beliefs or they rule you.

The mental TV monitor has been included in the exercise simply because many people spend a great deal of time watching television. Despite problems with TV over-viewing, the fact remains that, to a large extent, watching TV is a practical way to mentally anchor impressions in a viewer's mind. While the visualization exercise makes note of using natural sounds as a backdrop, feel free to interject whatever audio you find soothing and therapeutic.

During my research into ancient and modern healing practices, I uncovered a Raja Yoga lesson that I believe can provide you a head start toward recovery. This lesson uses the enlarged TV Monitor within the framework of the Visualization Technique, to promote personal growth and progress.

First, a simplified course in Raja Yoga is in order.

With regard to illness, Raja Yoga texts instruct the Initiate to fix into consciousness a picture of illness as a temporary part of you, not as the true "You." (Depending on your religious denomination, feel free to interchange the term "You," "Divine Self," "Holy Spirit" or "Divine Energy."). Yogic discipline suggests the Initiate regard the "You" as indestructible, the True Nature.

In Yogic thinking, the "Divine Self" ("Infinite Energy" or "Universal Consciousness") is an inner source of power that transcends and is independent of both mind and body. The Divine Self simply works through the mind and body. It is not mind. It simply uses the mind to think. It is not body. It merely uses the body as a container to function. Tapping into infinite source energy can bring about a spontaneous cosmic consciousness and healing experience. Like parting with luggage prior to boarding an airplane, graphically picturing your healed body on a TV Monitor sets aside bodily symptoms and negative beliefs as mere baggage—something external to "Divine Self."

The benefit of Raja Yoga to a patient with a life-threatening illness is to recognize the Divine Self as independent of body—

immortal, invulnerable, invincible. For simplicity and working purposes, I have included the Raja Yoga principle in the Visualization Technique in order to permit you to stand aside and examine negative imagery from a witnessing perspective in order to overthrow and transcend it.

The TV monitor simply enables you to stand apart from the part of you that perceives illness. In this respect, it helps disconnect your Divine Self from arousal of toxic "I am my body" or "I am my symptoms" thinking and feeling.

You are a conscious co-creator; a divine Self.

What's the purpose of the remote control? Did you notice your guide punched a channel marked "Future Event?" Think of this as your own Future Event Channel (FEC), similar in nature to NBC or ABC, but without commercials. The FEC is a critical component of the visualization process, because without hope of a better future, it's well-known the physical body can wither away. This is a simple but effective way to change your life experiences, by imagining the outcome you intensely desire and converting your strong intent and feeling into audible sound and visible light.

The questions your guide asks are pertinent. No one but you can dictate your life's purpose and what you've learned from crisis. These are important questions to consider. Perhaps you've learned to follow your natural abilities and instincts wherever they lead, realizing in this way, you're tuning into a universal frequency and Higher Power.

Critical Comments:

Let's review the basics. There are a few "must" back-to-wellness factors that those who suffer from seemingly incurable illnesses have found to be highly effective in the results-oriented visualization process. They are:

Healing Factor #1:

See your particular challenge as temporary.

Healing Factor #2:

Picture your natural killer cells neutralizing any cancer or virus-infected cells. "See" yourself fully restored to health.

Healing Factor #3:

Make sure you place great depth of feeling behind the mental impression you create. The greater the intensity of your mental imagery, the shorter its time to actualization.

Healing Factor #4:

Confidently picture your body in perfect health and harmony with all parts working flawlessly together.

Healing Factor #5:

Ask for guidance.

Healing Factor #6:

Note the dynamic life lesson(s) you've learned.

Healing Factor #7:

Mentally picture your new, selfless mission as already achieved.

Reminders:

To be effective, the visualization exercise requires three-a-day practice sessions or, quite literally, it wears off. After a week of regular three-a-day practice, feel free to merely go through a preliminary countdown and enter the Healing Temple directly.

Be patient. For your own comfort and well-being, allow an incubation period of at least thirty days to emotionally transcend past toxic beliefs and habitual thoughts so as to give birth to your new vision. Don't force yourself to achieve results. Allow events to unfold naturally as a result of your new practice. And always permit your physician to monitor your progress.

A condensed version of the visualization exercise:

The visualization exercise detailed below is yet another step-by-step program that can have a major impact on your ability to deal with a life-threatening illness, or virtually any crisis in your life. It's meant to supplement, not replace, allopathic medicine, though you should plan to practice it three times a day. Take a mental picture of the thymus gland (available at your local library) before you begin the exercise so the mental impressions you produce are clear in your mind. The following scenario is the internal image you want to see on your mind's eye.

Like a movie camera, take a mental snapshot of the thymus gland pouring out natural killer cells into your blood stream for one or two minutes.

For the next minute or two, imagine the natural killer cells in your blood stream turn to magnets neutralizing any abnormal cells in your body.

Repeat this process three times a day, in a slow, rhythmic way as the pictures you're envisioning become impressed on your mind.

Once you begin marshalling this powerful mind-body communication technique, it can protect your health without your ever being aware of the subtle changes taking place on all levels of your being.

Wellness Exercise #3:
The Prayer/Dream Exercise

The sleep state can be a powerful workshop for problem-solving, and knowledge of how to link it with simple prayer can help you to return to good health. After completing the Visualization Technique, plant a dream/prayer message in your subconscious (or use your mental screen surrounded by healing light) before going to bed. The self-dialogue model I use to convey a constructive back-to-wellness dream to my sleeping subconscious is as follows:

> *"Tonight I pray to Divine Spirit that my health will be restored completely, and I will form a dream that will hasten my total recovery. I pray to experience total restoration of my health in my dream that will materialize in my waking state as well."*

For more information on the nature of dreams, I recommned you consult one or both of these insightful studies: *Dreams That can Change Your Life* by Alan B. Siegel, Ph.D. and *The Dream and the Underworld* by James Hillman. Yet there is little available information on "seeding" or directing dreams to lead you into the wellness experience.

Sandra Ingerman, a psychologist who wrote *Welcome Home: Following Your Soul's Journey of Hope*, talks about attempting a nontraditional prayer and dream-healing approach after conventional medicine told her that her case was untreatable. She explained the alternative healing approach this way:

240

Every night before I went to sleep, I prayed for help in a dream. This was an act of desperation; nothing else that I knew of was helping. I asked diligently every night for months. One night I had the most extraordinary dream: I dreamed that I was in the living room of my house. Suddenly a young, handsome Native American appeared from behind my couch dressed in blue jeans and a blue work shirt. In his hand was a rattle made of an extraordinary skin that was translucent blue. He pointed his finger at the place in my body where I was experiencing pain and said, "You have a problem right here." He shook his rattle over the diseased part of my body. At that moment I could feel the pain lift out of my body. I knew inside the dream that I had had a healing and that I would be free of pain forever. The man disappeared at that point. Indeed, I did awaken from the dream pain-free and have been free of this problem ever since.

I was so impressed with Sandra Ingerman's suggestions that I have chosen to nightly use dream consciousness as a source of creative and back-to-wellness power, and I recommend that you do also. Better yet, buy and read her book, or visit Sandra's website at www.shamanicvisions.com. She can be contacted at P.O. Box 4757, Santa Fe, NM, 87502..

Wellness Exercise #4:
The Relaxation (De-Stressing) Strategy

This is an optional exercise to control stress. It allows you to reach beyond the invisible line between willpower and imagination. Here is how the relaxation exercise works:

Place yourself in a quiet and comfortable place where there is no interruption. If you wear glasses, remove them.

This will be a signal to your unconscious mind the session is about to begin.

During the day, sitting up in a comfortable chair is best. However, it's okay to lie down at night and conduct this exercise just before you fall asleep. (If used during a particular medical test, you may be lying either on your back or on your side.)

After you've practiced this exercise regularly, you'll find, as I did, it takes only a few minutes to get the outcome of physical and mental relaxation you're seeking. This observation is not based on any scientific fact; it is merely an inner realization—a direct experience you will "know."

Don"t close your eyes just yet. Place your hands on your lap. Then say to yourself very slowly:

I see my eyes roll up to the top of my head as high as they possibly can. While looking up, I try to keep my eyelids down. I take a deep breath, let the air out and close my eyes. I am becoming relaxed and calm, like gentle waves rolling off a remote island. I am starting to feel mentally and physically restful. I am now in a wonderful state of comfort.

From the top of my head to the tips of my toes, a wonderful mind and body communication takes place. Each breath I breathe brings in a wonderful sense of elation. I feel my body begin to harmonize and float into a remarkable state of relaxation.

My mind and my body breathe as one, together in a wonderful state of harmony.

I now begin to notice that above my head is a shining glow, like a white light radiating health and healing. The light is relaxing, soothing, and rejuvenating. As I count from three—back to one, this healing and relaxing energy of light will enter my body through the back of my head.
(Slowly) Three. Two. One.

(Slowly) I see Infinite Energy in the form of a white healing light, entering the back of my head. The light energy begins to navigate itself slowly down my body relaxing and healing everything it touches. I see a picture of the healing relaxing light slowly moving down my forehead. It is relaxing and healing all parts of my face and neck. My shoulders feel relaxed and completely comfortable. I see the light healing and relaxing everything in its path. It is penetrating every muscle, every cell of my body. The healing light is now flowing completely through my arms. Now I see it traveling through my hands. I now feel it pass through my torso. The healing and relaxing light is now tracking through my thighs. It is now moving smoothly through my legs. Now it is flowing through my feet.

I am completely relaxed from head to toe.

Every part of my body is now relaxed and healing. I am relaxing into a deeper, deeper state.

I now see my entire body totally wrapped in a protective covering, like a cocoon. I feel safe enveloped in this calm and healing cocoon of Infinite Energy enveloping my entire body. I am thoroughly surrounded and immersed in a relaxing and healing light. A relaxing light. A healing light. I see myself covered in the presence of this healing and relaxing light. Its healing and de-stressing energy is penetrating every muscle, every cell of my body.

Every muscle, every cell of my body is relaxed and enveloped in this healing and relaxing cocoon of Infinite Energy. I see myself relaxing and falling into an ever deeper and deeper state of relaxation.

I am completely relaxed and can now show no fear because of it. I feel secure. All of my muscles are at complete rest. I'm now completely and totally free of all tension, all anxiety, all fear.

Now I'm going to stop this part of the process and allow myself to notice how powerful my mind and body are. I'm observing my mind and my body and how they work together and how Infinite Energy is focused on relaxation and healing.

And now that I'm ready to let the healing light of Infinite Energy leave, I will simply shift my attention to what I am about to do next.

I'm feeling very, very renewed, self-empowered and immersed in healing energy. I'm shifting my attention with each moment that happens.

I'm now letting my eyes open very slowly. I'm stretching my muscles and looking around. I'm feeling exceptionally good. Very, very good.

I'm taking my time, shifting my attention. Stretching. Looking around. Letting feeling come back in my hands and body. I'm feeling very, very good.

If you have any pain during a particular medical test, here is what to say to yourself:

I now see a miniaturized version of (myself, my spouse, significant other, sports trainer, therapist, whomever) gently massaging and relaxing the area. I see the entire area in a thoroughly relaxed state. I see every atom and every cell in the area relaxing.

Each breath brings a powerful feeling of tranquility. The healing light of Infinite Energy moves in with power and comfort.

I'm doing well. I'm doing very well. My mind and my body are working together as one in a very focused, harmonious state.

I now see a very powerful interaction between my mind and body taking place.

And now, I'm going to stop this part of the process and notice how powerful my mind and body are. I'm observing my mind and body, how they breathe together, and how the energy is focused.

And when I'm ready to let the relaxing, healing light leave, I'll simply shift my attention to what I'm about to do next. Shifting my attention with each moment that takes place, I'll be feeling very, very renewed in energy. Letting my eyes open and look around when ready, I will feel very, very good.

NOTE: You can practice this exercise any time, any place. In a few brief minutes it will prepare you to face situations—a medical procedure, for example—without fear or anxiety.

Wellness Exercise #5:
The "Acting As If" Healing Strategy

Despite cancer, many of the long-term survivors I interviewed acted as if they were well—not only during the diagnostic process but also after years of relief. Yet I found it difficult to label this survival technique, since it really is a mode of thought and an ingrained behavior. I came up with the "Acting As if" title after reading *Act Now!* the marvelous book by Dale Anderson, M.D. that I have already mentioned several times. Dr. Anderson contends that patients can turn their medical condition around by acting as if they're healthy, even when they don't feel that way.

Wellness Exercise #6:
Optimizing the Present Moment to Heal

Two days you can't do anything about are yesterday and tomorrow. Your power to change and heal is only in the present moment. You must understand that today is the only place you can take aim to reach wellness. Like the philosopher Kierkegaard sagely observed,

> *We become what we think about. Life is a self-fulfilling prophecy. It can only be understood backwards, but it must be lived frontward.*

Still, some participants in the *Quiet Miracles* workshops fail to fully understand this important concept, and continue to focus their attention on past wounds and hurts. These same workshop participants often hope that by some miracle—without their taking an iota of responsibility for their medical journey and life—circumstances somehow will change for the better. On the other hand, the primary focus of those patients who do become long-term survivors is the moment at hand. Remember that the present moment is where change takes place, though change, once begun, may also influence both the past and the future. As Thomas Carlyle once said, "Our grand business is not to see what lies dimly at a distance but to do what lies clearly at hand."

Below is a chart that I use to get this important concept across. Grade yourself on where you are in terms of power or powerlessness at this moment in time by asking yourself, am I in:

- WHAT WAS

- WHAT WILL BE or,

- WHAT IS?

WHAT THOUGHTS DO YOU CHOOSE TO EMPOWER?

The Power of Choice!

I. WHAT WILL BE (Tomorrow)
Remaining in This Position Blocks Healing

- Worries about tomorrow cloud perception and diminish energy and healing.

- You can't move forward toward healing of mind, body, and spirit from this powerless position.

- Remaining in this state quite literally reduces the functioning of your body's defence mechanisms.

II. WHAT IS (Today—the Present Moment)
Your Optimum Power to Heal Yourself Is Here!

- Your maximum power to heal yourself is in the present moment.

- From this position you can claim your freedom of choice, effect change, form a new beginning, stretch your capabilities, and expand your life.

- Time doesn't stand still. It's ticking away this very minute, and the future is arriving right now. The present is all you have to work with to bring forth new opportunities for personal growth and healing.

- Since the present is quickly becoming what was, if you choose not to participate in it fully, you lose its potential to start anew.

- Step out of this position and you give your power away to I or III. The result: Personal and spiritual growth stops.

- Move out of this position to I or III, and you impede the functioning of your immune system.

III. WHAT WAS (Yesterday—the Past)
Remaining in This Position Blocks Healing

- This is a reactive, shrinking position that breeds negative thinking and feelings of victimization.

- If you abdicate the power of II to this position, you are bound to live in a state of powerlessness (e.g., hopelessness and helplessness).

- Expend too much energy in this mental position and you weaken the functioning of your immune system.

- If you're content to waste energy here, it will not be available for healing in II.

- Choose to remain here and you face each new day knowing the past has control over you and your life choices will be made for you. As a consequence, you will have little or no opportunity to grow and heal.

There's a wonderful poem entitled "I Am" that fits in perfectly with the above principles. I wish I knew the author. It goes like this:

> I was regretting the past
> > And fearing The Future...
> Suddenly, my Lord was speaking
> > "My Name is I Am"
> He paused . . .
> > I waited . . .

He continued "When you live
> In the past with its mistakes
> and regrets, it is hard —
> I am not there.

My name is not I was.

When you live in the future
> With its problems and fears,
> it is hard — I am not there.

My name is not I will be.

When you live in the moment
> it is not hard — I am here.
> My name is I Am.

Wellness Exercise #7:

Writing down what you want to enter your life as a real event.

1. Start by thinking and writing down in detail what you want to enter your life as a real event(s) in time and space.

2. Always practice with specific goals in mind.

3. Imagine and five-sense what you want to achieve as a completed event.

4. Don't be in a rush.

5. Once you can "see" and FEEL the outcome you want to achieve as a "given", "know" it's on its way to becoming yours and the practice session is over.

You look at life through the lens of your beliefs, thoughts, expectations, and feelings. If, for example, you choose to view life through a lens of unforgiveness, the pictures you'll see will be colored by that thought and feeling. The life experiences you'll attract to yourself will follow your thoughts and feelings. Put this principle to the test by monitoring your self-destructive beliefs, thoughts, and feelings for the next thirty days, while reflecting on the fact that what you presently observe is the consequence of your past beliefs, thoughts and feelings.

Better yet, make a binding contract with yourself that for the next thirty days, you'll carry around a little notebook, and each time you say or think,

"I think ..."

"I believe ..."

"I feel ..."

"This is how I see it, "

"It's my opinion that ..."

"I'm convinced that ..."

... write it down in a notebook. It won't be long before you'll see the connection between your interior and exterior life, the destructive influence of self-limiting thoughts, and the life events they attract. This exercise will prompt you to choose your thoughts very cautiously.

Once you've completed your list, make a separate copy and carry it around with you. Look at it several times a day, as a reminder that habitual beliefs and thoughts, like standing orders, are the rules you live by.

To begin a new way of thinking, and to turn your health and life around—write it down and— it will come.

Dr. Henriette Ann Klauser has written a truly extraordinary book entitled, *Write It Down, Make It Happen*. It should be in everyone's home library.

Dr. Klauser suggests that by writing down your fears, you begin the process of dispelling them. The idea, says Klauser, is to start a journal and add a "fears page" listing your present worries. If, for example, you write, "I'm just not good enough," then below this belief, on the same page write, in first person, present tense, the statement, "I'm the best," which diminishes the emotional charge of the fearful emotion.

Think outside your beliefs.

Your beliefs limit what you can experience. You need to think beyond your self-limiting beliefs. A new focus will take you outside the artificial boundaries of your current mode of thinking and feeling.

Dr. Klause is suggesting you "write through to resolution."

Each choice you make is creating your destiny. The idea is to keep writing and writing until you get to the point where you FEEL an emotional release of the particular drama into which you've looped your negative thinking and emotions. This exercise will tend to separate you from your toxic thoughts and feelings, which are limiting you from what you most want to experience.

When push comes to shove, it's all about going the extra mile.

Until you personally commit to going the extra distance to move out of fear, you'll never know if you can let loose from it or not. Someone once said, "Work your loom, choose your threads." Ralph Walso Emerson expressed it even better. "Do not go where the path may lead," he said, "go instead where there is no path and leave a trail."

Caveat: Don't stop writing until you get past the point of resistance that your current toxic thoughts and feelings have rigidly set. That, says, Dr. Klauser, is "often right past the place where you think you have run out of ideas or solutions."

Looking for change? Are you clear enough to commit your life to bringing change NOW?

Then, writing a daily list of thoughts and feelings you want to focus consciousness on is an absolute must.

Dr. Klauser suggests going beyond the outcome you're focusing your attention on. In addition to writing down in detail what you want to achieve, craft something like the following (below is an example I've used):

Every day in every way, I see myself perfectly healthy, because I have a wife, children and grandchildren who need my attention and my love. I also have workshop attendees who, to survive, need the information I have acquired.

Thinking this way gives me an electrifying jolt of joy regarding why I choose to see my goals and purposes already achieved. By continuing to think this way, you'll cause your mind to objectify and FEEL the energy shifting to health and well-being. And because of that, you'll FEEL immense joy. I complete the exercise by emotionally saying to myself, "So be it! YES!"

So why not start your "To-Be List" right here and right now? Getting what you want equates to keeping your eye (and feelings) on the prize. As an example to get you going, here's my personal "To-Be List" for this week:

- Remind myself I get to consciously choose what I focus on.
- Focus on and choose only good-feeling thoughts.
- Write at least 10 pages of a new book I'm working on.
- Put on a happy face and listen to agree rather than voice rigid opinions.
- Know that an outcome-oriented image backed by strong feelings and intention is stronger than an actual experience.
- Remind myself if I talk about illness, anger, etc., it causes my body to degenerate more.
- If I find myself locked into a particular fearful belief, ask myself. "What's the toxic thought causing me to feel or vibrate this way?"
- Expand and energize each present moment by staying out of past wounds and future worries.
- Only flow energy to what I want.
- Keep in mind that I grow the most under the greatest challenges.
- Search for new ways to make my Quiet Miracles workshops better and better.
- Remind myself that my life depends on my every thought and feeling and, if I think fear (vibrate it), it will come.
- Know inwardly if I don't perceive or energize what I want, I can't create it.

Next, write down whatever entrenched explanations you make to yourself for NOT taking action to monitor and change your self-destructive beliefs.

As you implant new, healthy thoughts and feelings of wellness in your mind, tell yourself:

No longer am I going to choose to live by old pessimistic beliefs that have been ruling my life. My new beliefs in total wellness are now under construction. As I shift my primary focus to imaging and feeling the best possible outcomes as "done deasl," without worrying about results, I'll get exactly what I focus my attention on.

Wellness Exercise #8:
The Post-It ™ Note Exercise.

In your office, home, car, room, or any other place where you can find privacy, sit down and ask yourself this question: "What do I want to achieve above all else?" Then, when you've settled on your goals, find several words that best describe your desire, which could be better health, more money, a better relationship and so on. Then, on Post-It™ notes, write the words you have chosen. Place the Post-It™ notes on your refrigerator, in your car, in your wallet or handbag, alongside your bed, or fasten one to a mirror. Put them anywhere you can't help but see them every day. The Post-It™ notes I use contain four words:

Every
Day
Way
Healthy

Using the above four words, I am pictorially and vividly telling myself by repeated self-suggestion: "Every day in every way I AM perfectly healthy." This is a *total outcome-oriented* exercise, so you want to . . .

Picture yourself as presently healthy!

In linking the Post-It® Note Exercise with your Visualization Exercise, The Suspension of Damaging Thoughts Technique, and the other approaches, you focus the energy of your thoughts and feelings to external manifestation. Remain persistent, and your mental images will manifest as an *anchored belief* of wellness. This strong belief will vibrationally activate the Law of Attraction, producing the desired matching event with powerful efficiency.

You can also use Post-It™ notes, or even small cards, to remind yourself of favorite quotations. You'll be amazed at how simple it is to implant peace-of-mind directly into the recesses of your subconscious mind.

Wellness Exercise #9:
The "Mirror" Technique

Practice this captivating exercise regularly, along with the other longevity tools described, and you'll quickly enhance the quality of your life while helping heal body, mind, emotions and spirit.

It's been said that Winston Churchill and other great orators used this mirror technique to prepare themselves before making speeches. However, you're seeking to send the powerful energy of your beliefs, mental images, and feelings to an audience of one: YOU. Get the message across to your subconscious mind and the results can be remarkable. This exercise strengthens your inner belief that you can, indeed, achieve the outcome you're visualizing.

Here's how The "Mirror" Technique works:

1. Stand in front of a mirror.

2. Pull in your stomach and keep your chest out.

3. Take three or four deep breaths.

4. Feel a sense of power rising up in your entire being.

5. Look into your eyes.

6. Watch your lips move and silently or out loud state in a positive tone: *"Every day in every way I AM perfectly healthy!"*

7. Let this phrase (mantra) pass through your mind several times and then dismiss it.

As you repeat the above exercises three times a day, you'll notice that along with a surge of new strength, *if you act the part—you become it!*

Wellness Exercise #10: The "Talking to Your Subconscious Mind" Strategy

Ordering your subconscious mind to carry out your directives is another potent longevity tool at your disposal. Here's a personal example of this "mental implantation" strategy in action. Recently, I was searching for a way to resolve a financial problem in regard to some work I was creating for a client. It entailed an enormous amount of extra effort, which he requested but for which he was unwilling to pay. It was quite disturbing, because I was losing significant revenue on the venture. So, I said to my subconscious,

"Look, I'm tired of trying to figure out a solution to this problem. I'm putting it in your hands. Find a solution ASAP, please." After a few hours, the solution popped into my mind. I would simply ask the client to sign off on a document, agreeing he is willing to pay me prior to any additional work he requests. To my complete surprise, he said, "Okay!" The growth lesson: "The way out is often the way through."

Here are several more examples of talking to your subconscious mind: To make sure you're not late for an important meeting, simply order your subconscious to remind you in advance. Or, if your muscles ache, command them to bring balance to your physical body. Or, if you're working on a new mental exercise, ask your subconscious mind to methodically get the job done, step-by-step. It's been my experience that you need to be crystal clear about the specific issue you're requesting your subconscious mind to resolve.

Wellness Exercise #11:
The Changing Beliefs Exercise

This is an adaptation of an excellent exercise described in my favorite book, *The Nature of Personal Reality* by Jane Roberts. This strategy is basically a form of self-hypnosis. For a period of three to four minutes each day, tell yourself the following:

> *For the next thirty days, I'll suspend any belief in illness and consciously accept a strong belief in wellness. I'll rehearse success by pretending I'm under hypnosis. I'll view myself as both the hypnotist and subject. For the next thirty days, I'll see no conflict between my present circumstance and my new belief. I'll pretend and feel as if the belief in wellness I imagine is mine entirely.*

Wellness Exercise #12:
Body under repair:
Immuno-self-therapy

When I begin to feel myself moving into a drama of despair, or if I'm wondering if, on deeper levels, a pattern of wellness is actually taking place, very quickly I say to myself, "My body is now under repair. Tremendous health-promoting change is taking place. Even though I may not as yet 'see' back-to-wellness changes actually taking place, they'll only take form if I *believe* and *feel* they can." I also practice repeating to myself, "Every day in every way, I'm perfectly healthy." The outcome is almost instant. I feel *as if* what I'm thinking, imagining and feeling is real(ity). This validating action—based purely on exuding a heightened belief in wellness—serves to generate even more optimistic imagery, thereby strengthening positive bodily conditions and a visceral sense of well-being.

Look at this practice as a game, as fun. Imagine and actually feel your health totally restored. Conjure up clear mental pictures of this condition. Remember "like attracts like" and with thoughts of recovery now mentally seeded and mapped out, chances are excellent your immune system will respond favorably.

Let me once again remind you of the powerful force behind all of the above exercises:

Every belief and mental picture backed with strong emotion, seeks to find inner and outer realization!

The above principle is the essence of my workshops.

**Learning as you go —
by creating your own personal wellness environment.**

Do your family and friends energize or de-energize you? Ever notice how you rarely see optimists hanging out with people who bring them down? On a personal note, I make it a daily practice to create an invigorating, controlled therapeutic reality that offers life-giving hope. I'm not specifically looking to surround myself with Pollyannas, but I'm really turned on by the positive energy created by vibrant people. At times such energy can be excessive and not heartfelt, but more often the flow of permeating energy emitted by upbeat people does feel good—like a revitalizing current.

A physical "miracle" first requires "seeing" a mental "miracle!"

Focusing on the positive is using the power of thought and feeling constructively. For this reason, I make it a hard-and-fast rule not only to focus on positive thoughts but to intersperse positive ideas into conversations I engage in, especially when the dialogue moves toward pessimistic discussions of life's problems. To continue otherwise is harmful to others as well as to yourself. Norman Vincent Peale, author of *The Power of Positive Thinking*, suggests we get in the habit of rooting out certain little negative statements that enter into our conversations and self-talk. For example, when Peale intimately analyzed his conversations, he noticed he was in the habit of making statements like, "I wonder if …." and, "I don't think I can do that." He concluded that the negative orientation of such commonplace phrases affects our mind in a harmful manner, psychologically lowering self-image and clouding our vision of life's possibilities. This is reason enough to change that picture and focus on making a private contract with yourself to

Only declare about your health the future probabilities you want to bring into your life.

Negative thoughts give birth to more of the same, which weakens your body. So, if you want to put the Law of Attraction to work for you in your life, it's a matter of asking yourself,

"Where do I choose to invest my energy?"

To put the same principle in a diiferent way, you might want to ask yourself, "Why would anyone consciously choose to surround themselves with:

- energy-draining people who are filled with self-doubt, lack optimism and initiative;
- people who believe they can not ordain their own destiny;
- those who choose to focus on life's de-energizing unhealthy situations, almost as if it were a sign of honor;
- people who unrelentingly visualize and generally talk about the negatives;
- those who constantly pursue and discuss dire news such as who died recently, the lurid details of the latest crime, etc.

Given a bank of limitless probable choices, why not choose to be with:

- People with vitality who turn adversity into advantage, such as long-term cancer survivors who have triumphed over crisis.
- "Action initiators" who understand fully that change requires forward action on their part.
- People who make it a habit to look for the seed of a solution that lies in seemingly insoluble challenges, as

well as the insightful life lessons required for spiritual development.

- Individuals who believe they can activate the Law of Attraction, thus creating the life circumstance they want to experience.
- Those who live their life with the fulfilling belief, "If it's meant to be, it's up to me!"
- Self-starters who live in the present, rather than reliving the past.

The secret of achieving on-going wellness and enriching your life is to place yourself on the road to predictable, long-term survival. It's asking yourself, "What future fearful events are likely to take place in my life based on my present thoughts, expectations and feelings?" It's learning to live in the present moment, where creativity can flourish, and *not having anything left of your candle when your life is over.* The message: Each day, light the candle.

In opening a new chapter of your life, give yourself the following three questions as a gift to draw upon for wisdom and knowledge:

#1: "Do you know what conscious choices brought you to where you are today?"

#2: "What would you attempt to do if you knew for sure you could not fail?"

#3: "From a field of infinite probable future events, what are you thinking into your life right here and right now?"

Henry David Thoreau once said, "Go confidently in the direction of your dreams! Live the life you've imagined."

Be assured it really is done unto you as you believe.

Your Daily Wellness Action Plan

"If you want a quality, act as if you already have it."
    – William James, M.D., Father of Psychology

You're now at The Tipping Point. It's time to make a conscious choice to either stay in the status quo and attract more of the same events into your life, or extend your boundaries to experience wellness.

Which will it be?

During my years working with long-term cancer survivors and workshop attendees, it has become evident to me that there are seven levels of awareness or soul growth that survivors pass through in the course of conquering a chronic illness. As you read through the list, please reflect seriously on each level, and ask yourself where the bulk of *your* mental energy is being focused. Read each level like your life actually depended on it. I believe it does. The effort you make to move on toward a new level of awareness may be the most important one you've ever made.

The first level of awareness

Individuals with a chronic illness *feel* like they're definitely "not going to make it."

They *believe* this must be so, and this belief engenders a feeling of hopelessness. And they will *continue* to feel this dispondency until they empower themselves to move beyond the belief that they're "not going to make it."

At this level of understanding, individuals have yet to see the connections between their mind and the functioning of their immune system. They're not yet aware that their beliefs, thoughts, and emotions affect their body's basic defense systems. They don't perceive that their body is under attack not only from countless abnormal cells but also from a daily barrage of their own negative beliefs. By the same token, they simply cannot convince themselves that a constructive set of beliefs can bring wellness to their body and positive events into their lives. Often, they find no meaning or sense of purpose in life, and this lack is mirrored in their physical condition and the tenor of their daily life.

The second level of awareness

As individuals move up to this level of consciousness, they're not yet receptive to the belief that life offers them multiple wellness alternatives, but they take the first step in self-realization by accepting that their beliefs and feelings *can* influence their health. They also come to realize that beliefs are not facts. They begin to understand that strong mental images communicate instantly with the cells in their body through molecular messengers. And, through daily practice of strategic back-to-wellness techniques, they begin to sense that positive belief, emotional intent, and mental imagery *can* influence their physical well-being. By expanding their focus, they become increasingly aware that the smallest mental or emotional thought can neurologically affect the functioning of their immune system, for good or for ill.

The third level of awareness

Individuals begin to grasp that life is truly a multiple choice quiz in which they can choose to alter, or refrain from altering, their mental response to chronic illness. Within their conscious attention, they become aware others have fought and beat life-threatening illnesses by taking control of their medical journey and life, and they begin to see the possibility that they can do the same through the power of belief and emotion. At this stage of consciousness, they become aware that focusing on thoughts and feelings of illness sets up adverse conditions that affect the functioning of their immune system. They sense if they don't find answers, they'll see the same outcome repeated over and over. They start the process of listening intently to their toxic self-talk, detecting that "maybe life really is an 'inside job.'" Through self-exploration, they learn the quantum notion that "there is no reality until it is perceived reality." Through thought-assessment they discover that the emotional lens through which they perceive life can dispense either wellness or illness energy waves, based solely on their personal attitude.

The fourth level of awareness

Individuals sense that by taking full responsibility to move their focus away from the emotional debris of past wounds and hurts, while remaining in the present moment, they can allow wellness to form a new and healthy physical reality. Viewing their immune system and life as one with their mental state, they recognize an inescapable truth—the inner mechanisms for healing reside unseen within the positive expectancy of their beliefs, thoughts, and feelings. Presented with hard data detailing multiple personality disorder, the placebo affect, the power of self-suggestion, the emotional and physical after-effects of the patient/doctor relationship, and how actors and actresses can alter the powerful biochemical nature of their body by their emotions, individuals with life-threatening illnesses begin to recognize it is entirely possible to consciously create a personal reality of wellness. At this level of consciousness, individuals wisely sense how harmful and limited in scope past destructive beliefs and thoughts are. They sense that they've been selling themselves short. They become more and more aware that they truly are conscious co-creators whose lives conform to their central beliefs and feelings.

The fifth level of awareness

At this level, individuals believe categorically that they are conscious co-creators of their own life experiences. They gain the inner realization to stop hindering their own incomparable powers to consciously create wellness, especially when meeting derisive cynicism. They view illness as a temporary rather than a permanent condition. Enlarging their focused beliefs, they embark on a true inner journey of wellness. They begin the process of examining and monitoring their harmful beliefs and feelings—their goal being to root out psychological or emotional issues they believe are the causative agents behind their illness. They sense intuitively that life demands growth on all levels—emotional, spiritual, and physical—and change comes not from without, but from within. Through regular practice of mental imaging, they understand clearly their life experiences are largely a consequence of their own highly emotional beliefs, expectations, and feelings. They continue to uncover how they've made themselves susceptible to illness, thereby suppressing the recuperative abilities of their immune system. Aware that they've been a prisoner of their own self-limiting beliefs, they divest themselves of those beliefs and begin to direct their positive regenerative energy toward health and growth.

The sixth level of awareness

Individuals become keenly aware that their optimum power to change their life is only in the present moment. At this level of consciousness, they make the deliberate choice to stop looking outward and turn inward for solutions to life's challenges. They regularly examine their subjective state of mind and willingly let go of self-pity and past de-energizing dramas and wounds. They direct their body's energy field daily to wellness in each ongoing present moment. They view life as a learning process of soul growth and development. They understand that at a deep level Ultimate Consciousness, of which they are a part, is an invisible reality that exists beyond the five senses and does not stop at the confines of their physical body.

The seventh level of awareness

Individuals "know" they're on this earth as conscious co-creators to learn to expand their awareness and create meaning and purpose in their lives. They "know" they can only create the goals they perceive; what they focus conscious intent and attention upon. They understand life is all about creating yourself. With greater clarity and intent, they see each crisis as a challenge. They recognize crisis as an opportunity to grow spiritually and enlarge the boundaries of their consciousness. Knowing they can not avoid the consequences of their self-limiting thoughts and feelings, they remain open to their inner voice and its intuitive directions. With openness and without prejudice, they mobilize their limitless energy as a conscious co-creator to form new habits of mind. They assess their life in each NOW moment, accepting total responsibility for their choices. If you are not now at this level of consciousness,

NOW is the time to begin forming a new wellness habit of mind.

NOW is the time to remove hidden emotional censors that delay the back-to-wellness process.

NOW is the time to form new positive mental habits.

NOW is the time to expand beyond your self-limiting boundaries.

NOW is the time to set aside past negative experiences.

NOW is the time to stay focused in the present moment.

NOW is the time to school yourself to engage your greater abilities as a conscious co-creator.

NOW is the time to build self-belief.

NOW is the time to energize your spirits to grow.

NOW is the time to take charge of your medical journey and life.

RIGHT NOW is the time to begin rehearsing success.

Your Back-to-Wellness
Daily Action Plan

Below is your back-to-wellness Daily Action Plan. It will aid you in taking charge of your medical journey—and life.

If the Daily Action Plan is persistently executed, you'll find firsthand a higher directing form of Supreme Intelligence assisting you—if you expect it will.

On Arising:

1. Practice the Outcome-Oriented Visualization Technique feeling the outcome you're mentally picturing as already achieved.

2. After practicing the Visualization Technique, ask yourself, "What positive experiences am I going to author today?" Mentally list them.

Ten-Minute Mid-Morning Break:

1. Practice the "White Healing Light" exercise.
2. Practice the "Changing Beliefs" exercise
3. Practice the "Talking to Your Subconscious Mind" exercise.

During the Day (as needed)

1. Note and list three self-defeating thoughts you send to yourself daily that cause you to feel sad and despondent. Whenever they arise, use the Suspension of Damaging Thoughts Technique with the affirming mantra, "Every day in every way, I AM perfectly healthy." Follow this with the "Changing Beliefs" exercise. If you're having difficulty with a specific self-destructive thought, dispute it. Follow this up by using the "Suspension of Damaging Thoughts" technique and the above life-affirming mantra.

2. Practice the Outcome-Oriented Visualization technique

3. Practice the Acting "As If" technique.

4. Play your favorite comedy tape for at least ten minutes to and from work.

5. Use the "Post-It Note®" exercise.

6. Practice the "Talking to Your Subconscious Mind" exercise.

7. Use the "Doodling Yourself to Wellness" exercise.

Fifteen-Minute Mid-Afternoon Break

1. Identify your personal life challenge (e.g. the central focus in your life) and look to resolve it.

2. Practice the "Mirror" technique

3. Practice the "Talking to Your Subconscious Mind" exercise

On Retiring

1. Prior to sleep each night, practice the Outcome-Oriented Visualization Technique.

2. Upon completion of the visualization technique, suggest to yourself you'll have a dream that'll resolve a specific personal challenge you're dealing with, e.g., "Tonight, I will dream that every day, in every way, I am perfectly healthy."

Let the advice of the following highly-respected sources be your ultimate back-to-wellness guide:

"*It matters if you don't just give up,*" said Stephen Hawking.

Louis Pasteur offered much the same advice when he stated, "*Let me tell you the secret that has led me to my goal. My strength lies solely in my tenacity.*"

A Japanese proverb expresses a similar thought: "*Fall seven times, stand up eight.*"

Sir Winston Churchill's clear focus was even more succinct: "*Never run away from anything. Never!*"

Further Reading

Jane Roberts – *The Nature of Personal Reality*

Roger Penrose, Ph.D. – *The Emperor's New Mind*

Amit Goswami, Ph. D. – *The Self-Aware Universe*

Lynda Madden Dahl – *The Wizards of Consciousness*

Nick Herbert, Ph.D. – *Quantum Reality*

Ervin Laszlo – *Science and the Akashic Field*

Professor Richard Wolfson – *Einstein's Relativity & the Quantum Revolution*

Brian Greene, Ph.D. – *The Elegant Universe*

Norman Friedman – *Bridging Science and Spirit*

David R. Hawkins, M.D., Ph.D. – *Power vs. Force*

Gerald Epstein, M.D. – *Healing Visualizations*

Martin Seligman, Ph.D. – *Learned Optimism*

Claude Bristol – *The Magic of Believing*

Sandra Ingerman, M.A., C.S.C. – *Soul Retrieval: Mending: the Fragmented Self*

Gary E. Schwartz, Ph.D. – *The Living Energy Universe*

Melvin Morse, MD – *Where God Lives*

Lynne McTaggart – *The Field*

Gary Schwartz, Ph.D. – *The Afterlife Experiments*

Bruce Lipton, Ph.D. – *The Biology of Complementary Medicine*

William James, Ph.D. – *The Varieties of Religious Experience*

Ernest Lawrence Rossi, Ph.D. – *The Psychology of Mind-Body Healing*

Margaret Talbot – "The Placebo Prescription" (*N.Y. Times Magazine*, 1/9/00)

Michael Crichton, M.D. – *Travels*

Richard Gerber, M.D. – *Exploring Vibrational Medicine*

Peter Russell – *From Science to God*

Brian Weiss, M.D. – *Messages From the Masters*

Shafica Karagulla, M.D. – *The Chakraas and the Human Energy Fields*

Carolyn Myss, Ph.D. – *Why People Don't Heal*

Candace Pert, Ph.D. – *Molecules of Emotion*

Robert Becker, M.D. – *The Body Electric*

Neale Donald Walsch – *A Conversation with God and The New Revelations*

Dale Anderson, M.D. – *Act Now*

Ostrander & Dchroeder – *Super-Learning 2000*

Edward E. Beal – *The Inner Secret*

Emile Coue, M.D. – *Conscious Autosuggestion*

Jane Roberts – *The Individual and Mass Events*

Jess Sterns – *The Sleeping Prophet*

Judith Orloff, M.D. – *Second Sight*

Carolyn Myss, Ph.D. – *Anatomy of the Spirit*

Larry Dossey, M.D. – *Healing Words*

Bennett G. Braun, M.D. – *Psychophysiology Phenomena in Multiple Personality*

Hall, O'Grady, Calandra, Ph.D – *Advances: The Journal of Mind-Body Health*

Victor S. Frankl, M.D. – *Man's Search for Meaning*